Preventive Medicine and Public Health

PreTest®
Self-Assessment
and Review

Preventive Medicine and Public Health

PreTest®
Self-Assessment
and Review

Sixth Edition

Edited by

Thomas B. Newman, M.D., M.P.H.
Assistant Professor of Pediatrics and of Epidemiology and Biostatistics
University of California, San Francisco

Warren S. Browner, M.D., M.P.H.
Assistant Professor of Epidemiology and Biostatistics and of Medicine
University of California, San Francisco

With the contributions of

Jack Percelay, M.D., M.P.H.

Robin Duryée, R.N., M.S.

McGraw-Hill, Inc.
Health Professions Division/PreTest® Series
New York   St. Louis   San Francisco   Auckland
Bogotá   Caracas   Lisbon   London   Madrid
Mexico   Milan   Montreal   New Delhi   Paris
San Juan   Singapore   Sydney   Tokyo   Toronto

4 5 6 7 8 9 0   DOCDOC   9 8 7 6 5 4

ISBN 0-07-051990-0

The editors were Gail Gavert and Bruce MacGregor.
The production supervisor was Clara B. Stanley.
R.R. Donnelley & Sons was printer and binder.
This book was set in Times Roman by R.J. Landi Book Production.

Library of Congress Cataloging-in-Publication Data

Preventive medicine and public health : PreTest self-assessment and
  review. -- 6th ed. / edited by Thomas B. Newman, Warren S. Browner.
    p.   cm.
  Rev. ed. of: Epidemiology and public health, 5th ed. c1989.
  Includes bibliographical references.
  ISBN 0-07-051990-0
    1. Public health -- Examinations, questions, etc.   2. Epidemiology -
  -Examinations, questions, etc.   3. Medicine, Preventive -
  -Examinations, questions, etc.   I. Newman, Thomas B.   II. Browner,
  Warren S.   III. Title: Epidemiology and public health.
    [DNLM: 1. Epidemiology -- examination questions.   2. Public Health-
  -examination questions.   WA 18 P9445]
  RA430.E65 1991
  362.1′076 -- dc20
  DNLM/DLC
  for Library of Congress   90-13702
                                                                      CIP

Contents

Preface

This sixth edition of *Preventive Medicine and Public Health: PreTest® Self-Assessment and Review* marks our third time as editors. One of our goals has been to make each edition an improvement over the last. We would greatly appreciate any suggestions from readers that might help us with that goal. Were there any topics covered on the board examinations for which you felt unprepared? Have some topics in this PreTest® been overemphasized? If you could choose them, which questions and answers would you delete or revise (why?) and which should be kept? Do you know any good epidemiology or biostatistics jokes? We would love to get mail from readers.

Thomas B. Newman, M.D., M.P.H.
Warren S. Browner, M.D., M.P.H.
74 New Montgomery St., Suite 600
San Francisco, CA 94105

Introduction

Preventive Medicine and Public Health: PreTest® Self-Assessment and Review, 6th Ed., has been designed to provide medical students, as well as physicians, with a comprehensive and convenient instrument for self-assessment and review within the field of epidemiology and public health. The 500 questions provided have been designed to parallel the format of the questions contained in Comprehensive Part II of the National Board of Medical Examiners examinations, the Federation Licensing Examination (FLEX), and the Foreign Medical Graduate Examination in the Medical Sciences (FMGEMS). This book will continue to be a useful study tool for Step 2 of the United States Medical Licensing Examination (USMLE).

Each question in the book is accompanied by an answer, a paragraph explanation, and a specific page reference to either a current journal article, a textbook, or both. A bibliography that lists all the sources used in the book follows the last chapter.

Perhaps the most effective way to use this book is to allow yourself one minute to answer each question in a given chapter; as you proceed, indicate your answer beside each question. By following this suggestion, you will be approximating the time limits imposed by the board examinations previously mentioned.

When you practice your examination-taking skills with this PreTest®, one way to maximize your score is to go through, answer all the questions you find easy, and skip over the more difficult ones initially. We do recommend, however, that once you come back to the more difficult questions, you spend as much time as you need to. You will then be more likely to retain the information. DO NOTE: When it comes to your examination for the board, you will do better to answer each question as you come to it and *not* skip around. Do not spend too much time on any one problem. Make a guess, circle the question, and come back to it. Otherwise, you can waste time looking on the computer score sheets for the question numbers you skipped or—the ultimate tragedy—you may discover that you forgot to skip a question and all your answers are off by one or more and time is running out.

When you have finished answering the questions in a chapter, you should then spend as much time as you need verifying your answers and carefully reading the explanations. Although you should pay special attention to the explanations for the questions you answered incorrectly, you should read every explanation. The authors of this book have designed the explanations to reinforce and supplement the information tested by the questions. If, after reading the explanations for a given chapter, you feel you need still more information about the material covered, you may wish to consult the references indicated.

Preventive Medicine and Public Health

PreTest®
Self-Assessment
and Review

Biostatistics and Methods of Epidemiology

DIRECTIONS: Each question below contains five suggested responses. Select the **one best** response to each question.

1. Epidemiology can be defined as the study of

(A) the etiology of disease in humans
(B) the frequency of causes of death in humans
(C) the determinants of frequency of disease in humans
(D) the distribution and determinants of frequency of disease in humans
(E) the patterns of organization and financing of health care

2. A sample of 1,000 people includes 120 who are hearing-impaired and 50 who are diabetic. If the number who are both diabetic and hearing-impaired is 6, then which of the following is true?

(A) Diabetes and hearing impairment appear to be independent characteristics
(B) Diabetics appear to be protected from hearing impairment
(C) Diabetics appear to be at greater risk of hearing impairment
(D) There is an interaction between diabetes and hearing impairment
(E) There is insufficient information to make any of the statements above

3. A measure of the amount of variation of a set of values about the mean is the

(A) regression coefficient
(B) standard error of the mean
(C) standard deviation
(D) range
(E) correlation coefficient

4. The association between low birth weight and maternal smoking during pregnancy can be studied by obtaining smoking histories from women at the time of the prenatal visit and then subsequently correlating birth weight with smoking histories. What type of study is this?

(A) Clinical trial
(B) Cross-sectional
(C) Cohort (prospective)
(D) Case-control (retrospective)
(E) None of the above

5. An investigator wishes to perform a randomized clinical trial to evaluate a new beta blocker as a treatment for hypertension. To be eligible for the study, subjects must have a resting diastolic blood pressure of at least 90 mmHg. One hundred patients seen at the screening clinic with this level of hypertension are recruited for the study and make appointments with the study nurse. When the nurse obtains their blood pressure 2 weeks later, only 65 of them have diastolic blood pressures of 90 mmHg or more. The most likely explanation for this is

(A) spontaneous resolution
(B) regression toward the mean
(C) baseline drift
(D) measurement error
(E) Hawthorne effect

6. Reye syndrome is an acute encephalopathy of childhood, accompanied by fatty infiltration of the liver. It has been linked to use of aspirin during infections with chickenpox or influenza. Children commonly progress through a sequence of stages that are used to grade severity and prognosis. If 30 percent of children progress only to stage I, 40 percent only to stage II, 20 percent only to stage III, and 10 percent to stage IV, what is the probability that a child will progress to stage IV, once that child has already reached stage II?

(A) 10 percent
(B) 14 percent
(C) 30 percent
(D) 33 percent
(E) None of the above

7. A study is undertaken to determine whether use of Newman and Browner's *PreTest Self-Assessment and Review* reduces sexual dysfunction related to anxiety before board examinations. One group of students studying for their board examinations was given the book to read; the other was not. The results are as follows:

Outcome	Got Book	Did Not Get Book
Sexual dysfunction	3	34
No sexual dysfunction	61	32

All the following statements are true EXCEPT

(A) these data could be analyzed using the chi-square test
(B) about half of the control group experienced sexual dysfunction
(C) unless one knows on what basis group assignment was made (i.e., randomized or not), the results are difficult to interpret
(D) the difference is probably due to chance
(E) a t test is inappropriate to analyze the data because the variables are categorical rather than continuous

8. Which of the following measures is used frequently as a denominator to calculate the incidence rate of a disease?

(A) Number of cases observed
(B) Number of new cases observed
(C) Number of asymptomatic cases
(D) Person-years of observation
(E) Persons lost to follow-up

9. If the chance of acquiring serologic evidence of human immunodeficiency virus (HIV) from an infected
sexual partner is a constant 30 percent
per year, what is the approximate
chance of becoming infected within 3
years?

(A) 10 percent
(B) 30 percent
(C) 66 percent
(D) 90 percent
(E) None of the above

10. In 1971, the crude birth rate in the
United States was approximately 17
per 1,000 population; the death rate
was 10 per 1,000; and the net in-
migration rate was 2 per 1,000. What
was the net growth rate per 1,000?

(A) 5
(B) 7
(C) 9
(D) 15
(E) 25

11. In nine families surveyed, the
numbers of children per family were 4,
6, 2, 2, 4, 3, 2, 1, and 7. The mean,
median, and mode numbers of children
per family are, respectively,

(A) 3.4, 2, 3
(B) 3, 3.4, 2
(C) 3, 3, 2
(D) 2, 3.5, 3
(E) none of the above

Questions 12–14

The results of a study of the incidence of pulmonary tuberculosis in a village in India are given in the table below. All persons in the village are examined during two surveys made 2 years apart, and the number of new cases was used to determine the incidence rate.

Category of Household at First Survey	Number of Persons	Number of New Cases
With culture-positive case	500	10
Without culture-positive case	10,000	10

12. What is the incidence of new cases per 1,000 person-years in households that had a culture-positive case during the first survey?

(A) 0.02
(B) 0.01
(C) 1.0
(D) 10
(E) 20

13. What is the incidence of new cases per 1,000 person-years in households that did not have a culture-positive case during the first survey?

(A) 0.001
(B) 0.1
(C) 0.5
(D) 1.0
(E) 5.0

14. What is the relative risk of acquiring tuberculosis in households with a culture-positive case compared with households without tuberculosis?

(A) 0.05
(B) 0.5
(C) 2.0
(D) 10
(E) 20

15. During the investigation of an outbreak of food poisoning at a summer camp, food histories were obtained from all campers as indicated in the table below. Which of the food items was probably responsible for the outbreak?

		Proportion Ill (Percent)	
	Food	Campers Who Ate Specified Food	Campers Who Did Not Eat Specified Food
(A)	Hamburger	61	48
(B)	Potatoes	70	35
(C)	Ice cream	40	50
(D)	Chicken	73	10
(E)	Lemonade	20	45

16. Which of the following statements concerning statistical inference is correct?

(A) If the p value = 0.05, then there is a 5 percent probability that the null hypothesis is true
(B) The null hypothesis generally states that there is a difference between the groups
(C) If the p value is greater than alpha, the null hypothesis is not rejected
(D) Knowledge of the sampling method is not important in determining statistical significance
(E) None of the above

17. In the study of the cause of a disease, the essential difference between an *experimental* study and an *observational* study is that in the experimental investigation

(A) the study is prospective
(B) the study is retrospective
(C) the study and control groups are of equal size
(D) the study and control groups are selected on the basis of history of exposure to the suspected causal factor
(E) the investigators determine who is and who is not exposed to the suspected causal factor

Questions 18–19

About 1 percent of boys are born with undescended testes. To determine whether prenatal exposure to tobacco smoke is a cause of undescended testes in newborns, the mothers of 100 newborns with undescended testes and 100 newborns whose testes had descended were questioned about smoking habits during pregnancy. The study revealed an odds ratio of 2.6 associated with exposure to smoke, with 95 percent confidence intervals from 1.1 to 5.3.

18. Which of the following statements is true?

(A) The odds ratio could be falsely elevated by the inclusion of infants whose testes were descended (but retractile) in the case group (misclassification bias)
(B) The odds ratio would be falsely reduced if parents of affected infants were more likely to remember or report their smoking (recall bias)
(C) Because the cases are newborns, but the exposure data came from their mothers, this is not a true case-control study
(D) Since the study was not blinded, it is impossible to rule out a placebo effect
(E) None of the above

19. Which of the following statements is true?

(A) The results provide no evidence that maternal cigarette smoking is associated with undescended testes in the offspring
(B) If the study results are accurate, they suggest that a baby boy whose mother smoked is about 2.6 times as likely to be born with testes undescended as a baby boy whose mother did not smoke
(C) The fact that the confidence interval excludes 1.0 indicates that $p > 0.05$
(D) The 90 percent confidence interval for these results would probably include 1.0
(E) None of the above

---

20. The probability of being born with condition A is 0.10 and the probability of being born with condition B is 0.50. If conditions A and B are independent, what is the probability of being born with either condition A or condition B (or both)?

(A) 0.05
(B) 0.40
(C) 0.50
(D) 0.55
(E) 0.60

21. All the following are important steps in decision analysis EXCEPT

(A) construction of a decision tree
(B) estimation of probabilities at chance nodes
(C) assignment of utilities
(D) estimation of sample size
(E) determination of how changes in probability estimates affect the decision

22. In order to determine the relationship between serum levels of sodium and antidiuretic hormone (ADH) in patients who have meningitis, the most appropriate study design would be

(A) repeated measurement of sodium and ADH in a patient with meningitis
(B) measurement of both sodium and ADH in a set of patients with meningitis
(C) measurements of sodium in one set of patients and of ADH in a different set of patients
(D) measurements of ADH in a set of patients with meningitis and a set of controls with other illnesses
(E) none of the above

23. All the following statements regarding the normal (Gaussian) distribution are true EXCEPT

(A) the mean = median = mode
(B) about 95 percent of observations fall within 2 standard deviations of the mean
(C) approximately 68 percent of observations fall within 1 standard deviation of the mean
(D) the number of observations between 0 and 1 standard deviation from the mean is the same as the number between 1 and 2 standard deviations from the mean
(E) the shape of the curve does not depend on the value of the mean

Questions 24–26

Lou Stewells, a pioneer in the study of diarrheal disease, has developed a new diagnostic test for cholera. When his agent is added to the stool, the organisms develop a characteristic ring around them. (He calls it the "Ring-Around-the-Cholera" [RAC] test.) He performs the test on 100 patients known to have cholera and 100 patients known not to have cholera with the following results:

	Cholera	No Cholera
RAC test +	91	12
RAC test –	9	88
Totals	100	100

24. All the following statements about the RAC test are correct EXCEPT

(A) the sensitivity of the test was about 91 percent
(B) the specificity of the test was about 12 percent
(C) the false negative rate was about 9 percent
(D) the predictive value of a positive result cannot be determined from the information above
(E) the predictive value of a negative result cannot be determined from the information above

25. Dr. Stewells next performs the test on 1,000 patients admitted to the hospital with profuse diarrhea. The results are as follows:

	Cholera	No Cholera
RAC test +	312	79
RAC test –	31	578
Totals	343	657

Which of the following statements is correct?

(A) The predictive value of a positive result is 312/343
(B) The predictive value of a positive result is 79/312
(C) The predictive value of a negative result is 578/(578 + 31)
(D) The incidence rate of cholera in this population is 343/1,000
(E) None of the above

26. After many years and dozens of publications, the RAC test achieves widespread acceptance, and Dr. Stewells' position in the Diarrhea Hall of Fame seems assured. However, with improvements in hygiene, the prevalence of cholera gradually falls from the high of about 35 percent of hospitalized diarrhea patients to only 5 percent. Which of the following statements about the effect of this fall in prevalence is true?

(A) The change in prevalence will reduce the predictive value of a negative result
(B) The predictive value of a positive result will decline
(C) The specificity of the test is likely to decline
(D) The specificity of the test will increase at the expense of its sensitivity
(E) None of the above

27. Randomization is a procedure used for assignment or allocation of subjects to treatment and control groups in experimental studies. Randomization ensures

(A) that assignment occurs by chance
(B) that treatment and control groups are alike in all respects except treatment
(C) that bias in observations is eliminated
(D) that placebo effects are eliminated
(E) none of the above

28. In comparing the difference between two means, the value of p is found to be 0.60. The correct interpretation of this result is

(A) the null hypothesis is rejected
(B) the difference is statistically significant
(C) the difference occurred by chance
(D) the difference is compatible with the null hypothesis
(E) sampling variation is an unlikely explanation of the difference

29. In a study of the cause of lung cancer, patients who had the disease were matched with controls by age, sex, place of residence, and social class. The frequency of cigarette smoking was then compared in the two groups. What type of study was this?

(A) Cohort (prospective)
(B) Case-control (retrospective)
(C) Clinical trial
(D) Historical cohort
(E) None of the above

30. The relationship between urinary tract infection (UTI) and lack of circumcision may be causal. Studies have also suggested that the relative risk for UTI in uncircumcised male infants is about 10. Which of the following is a valid implication of this observation?

(A) In male infants with fever, the yield of a urine culture is likely to be higher if the boy is circumcised

(B) In male infants in whom a UTI is documented but no abnormalities are detected on physical examination, the yield of urinary tract imaging to look for congenital urologic malformations (which predispose to UTI) is likely to be much higher if the infant is uncircumcised

(C) All male infants should be circumcised to prevent UTI

(D) If the association is causal, about 90 percent of UTIs in uncircumcised male infants are due to the fact that these infants are uncircumcised

(E) None of the above

Questions 31–33

Smoking and alcohol use are both risk factors for esophageal cancer. The hypothetical table below shows how the incidence of esophageal cancer varies with either smoking or alcohol use (but not both):

	Incidence (cases/10,000 person-yr)	
	Nonsmoker	Smoker
Nondrinker	10	50
Drinker	30	X

31. All the following statements are true EXCEPT

(A) in nonsmokers, the excess risk of esophageal cancer from drinking is 20 cases per 10,000 person-years

(B) in nondrinkers, the relative risk of esophageal cancer from smoking is 5.0

(C) the overall relative risk for smoking cannot be determined without knowledge of X and the proportion of the population that drinks

(D) the table shows that smoking causes more cases of esophageal cancer in this population than does drinking

(E) in nondrinkers, the excess risk of esophageal cancer from smoking is 40 cases per 10,000 person-years

32. If smoking and alcohol act independently to cause esophageal cancer under an *additive* model, what would be the expected value of X?

(A) 60
(B) 70
(C) 80
(D) 150
(E) None of the above

33. If smoking and alcohol act independently according to a *multiplicative* model, what would be the expected value of X?

(A) 70
(B) 80
(C) 120
(D) 1500
(E) None of the above

---

34. In the table below, data are presented on the number of children suffering from acute leukemia who were admitted to a hospital between 1970 and 1984. Correct conclusions about the data include which of the following?

Age (years)	Number of Children Admitted in Interval		
	1970–74	1975–79	1980–84
0–4	12	23	31
5–9	8	17	36
10–14	10	7	4
Total	30	47	71

(A) The incidence rate of leukemia decreased in children 10 to 14 years old
(B) The prevalence rate of leukemia increased in children between 1970 and 1984
(C) The incidence rate of leukemia increased in children 5 to 9 years old
(D) The number of children 9 years old and under admitted to the study hospital because of acute leukemia increased between 1970 and 1984
(E) None of the above

35. The Coronary Drug Project was a randomized trial to evaluate the efficacy of several lipid-lowering drugs. The 5-year mortality of the men who adhered to the regimen of clofibrate (i.e., took 80 percent of their medicine or more) was 15 percent; among those assigned to the clofibrate group who were less compliant, it was 24.6 percent. The result was highly statistically significant (p = 0.0001). From this one can conclude

(A) clofibrate was very beneficial to the patients who took it reliably
(B) clofibrate is not effective unless patients take at least 80 percent of the recommended doses
(C) either clofibrate or something associated with taking it reliably is strongly associated with reduced total mortality
(D) there was a problem with blinding in this study
(E) none of the above

36. The *attributable risk* of a disease estimates the maximum proportion of the disease in the population attributable to a particular risk factor. For example, in the U.S. the attributable risk of lung cancer from active smoking is about 85 percent; this means that active smoking may explain up to 85 percent of the cases of lung cancer that occur in the U.S. For a particular disease and risk factor, the attributable risk depends on

(A) the size of the population of interest
(B) the prevalence of the disease
(C) the relative risk (risk ratio) of the disease associated with the risk factor
(D) the duration of the disease
(E) none of the above

37. A randomized, double-blinded trial finds that oral corticosteroids are superior to placebo in hastening the resolution of otitis media with effusion. Possible reasons why this study might have given a falsely positive result include

(A) the sample size may have been too small
(B) the apparent effect might be a result of chance
(C) it may be difficult to determine accurately which effusions have resolved, which will lead to errors in determining the outcome of the study
(D) lax inclusion criteria may have led to inclusion of some subjects in the study who did not really have otitis media with effusion
(E) none of the above

38. Correct statements concerning statistical inference include which one of the following?

(A) If the p value is very low, the difference between the groups must be very large
(B) The standard error of the mean is used to estimate how closely the mean of a sample approximates the true population mean
(C) If the sample size is large enough, it is easy to achieve statistical significance at the 0.05 level, even when there is no difference between the groups
(D) Use of one-tailed rather than two-tailed tests of statistical significance will less often lead to rejecting the null hypothesis when it is true
(E) None of the above

39. An investigator is designing a randomized clinical trial to see whether vitamin E will prevent cancer in smokers. Which of the following is the LEAST important consideration in planning the sample size for the study?

(A) The expected incidence of cancer in the placebo group
(B) The frequency with which subjects are likely to be lost to follow-up or die from noncancer causes over the duration of the study
(C) The prevalence of smoking in the population
(D) The values for alpha and beta, the type 1 and type 2 error rates
(E) The magnitude of the preventive effect that the investigator wishes to be able to detect

Questions 40–41

The following questions refer to the receiver operating characteristic (ROC) curves for three different diagnostic tests (labeled 1, 2, and 3) shown below.

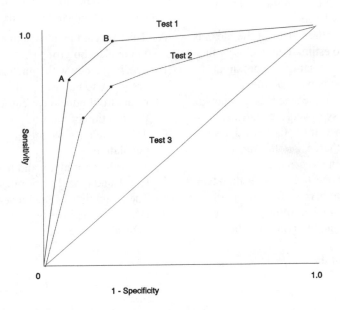

40. Which of the following statements about the figure is true?

(A) Test 2 is more sensitive than test 1
(B) Test 3 is totally useless
(C) If it is particularly important to avoid a false positive result, test 2 is preferable to test 1
(D) Test 3 performs perfectly
(E) None of the above

41. Which of the following statements about points A and B is correct?

(A) A and B are two different patients *with* disease on whom test 1 was performed
(B) A and B are two different patients *without* disease on whom test 1 was performed
(C) A and B represent varying thresholds for considering the result of test 1 to be indicative of disease
(D) If false negative results are to be avoided, point A represents the best choice
(E) None of the above

42. In a study of level of blood lead as a predictor of IQ in children, a simple linear regression analysis is performed. The regression coefficient for lead is -0.1 IQ points per μg Pb/dL blood. The coefficient is highly significant statistically ($p < 0.001$). Correct conclusions include which of the following?

(A) All else being equal, the expected difference in IQ between two children whose lead levels differ by 50 μg/dL is about 5 points
(B) The relationship between blood lead and IQ is linear
(C) Lead causes a decrease in the IQ in children of about 0.1 point for each μg/dL of blood lead
(D) The study provides convincing evidence that lead and IQ are independently associated
(E) None of the above

43. The prevalence of HLA-B27 among North American whites is 7 percent; among white American patients with ankylosing spondylitis, the prevalence of HLA-B27 is 90 percent. This indicates that

(A) the prevalence of ankylosing spondylitis is 0.7 percent
(B) the prevalence of ankylosing spondylitis is 6.3 percent
(C) the relative prevalence of ankylosing spondylitis associated with HLA-B27 is greater than 100
(D) the relative prevalence of ankylosing spondylitis associated with HLA-B27 is about 13
(E) the relative prevalence of ankylosing spondylitis associated with HLA-B27 cannot be estimated

44. All the following statements about life expectancy in the U.S. are true EXCEPT

(A) less than half of all deaths occur by age 75 years
(B) a 65-year-old woman can expect to live about 19 more years
(C) on average, women live about 7 years longer than men
(D) most of the increase in life expectancy since 1900 has been a result of decreasing rates of coronary heart disease
(E) if mortality does not change in his or her lifetime, a child born today will live an average of 75 years

45. True statements concerning cohort studies include all the following EXCEPT

(A) cohort studies are longitudinal in design
(B) subjects are selected on the basis of characteristics present before the onset of the condition being studied
(C) subjects are observed over time to determine the frequency of occurrence of the condition under study
(D) cohort studies can be retrospective
(E) cohort studies are necessary to estimate the prevalence of diseases

Questions 46–49

A research team wishes to investigate a possible association between smokeless tobacco use and oral lesions among professional baseball players. At spring training camp, they ask each baseball player about current and past use of smokeless tobacco, cigarettes, and alcohol, and a dentist notes the type and extent of the lesions in the mouth.

46. What type of study is this?

(A) Case-control
(B) Cross-sectional
(C) Cohort
(D) Clinical trial
(E) None of the above

47. After the players have been questioned about smokeless tobacco use and examined for lesions of the mouth, the data on the 146 players are tabulated as follows:

	Mouth Lesions	No Lesions	Total
User	80	30	110
Nonuser	2	34	36
Total	82	64	146

In this study, what is the incidence rate of mouth lesions among the baseball players who use smokeless tobacco?

(A) 80/30
(B) 80/110
(C) 82/146
(D) 30/110
(E) Cannot be calculated from the data given

48. All the following statements about the association between smokeless tobacco use and oral lesions in this study are true EXCEPT

(A) the odds ratio is $(80 \times 34)/(2 \times 30) = 45.3$
(B) smokeless tobacco users are about 45.3 times as likely as nonusers to have oral lesions
(C) the prevalence of smokeless tobacco use in this sample is 110/146
(D) the results are likely to be statistically significant
(E) the statistical significance could be calculated using a chi-square test

49. If the association between smokeless tobacco use and oral lesions in the last question is causal, approximately what proportion of the mouth lesions in the smokers are due to smokeless tobacco use?

(A) 27 percent
(B) 50 percent
(C) 73 percent
(D) 92 percent
(E) 99 percent

50. For many diagnostic or screening tests, there is a tradeoff between sensitivity and specificity. True statements include which of the following?

(A) Sensitivity would be extremely important when testing for amyotrophic lateral sclerosis (ALS) because there is no good treatment for it
(B) Because hypothyroidism in infancy is devastating if missed, a screening test for it should be highly specific
(C) Specificity is more important than sensitivity for screening tests
(D) In evaluating the potential usefulness of a screening test, the effectiveness of treatment for the disease screened for is important
(E) None of the above

51. The occurrence of a group of illnesses of similar nature at a rate above the expected number is called

(A) hyperendemic
(B) epidemic
(C) endemic
(D) enzootic
(E) pandemic

52. The time interval between entry of an infectious agent into a host and the onset of symptoms is called

(A) the communicable period
(B) the incubation period
(C) the preinfectious period
(D) the noncontagious period
(E) the decubation period

53. A randomized trial shows that a new thrombolytic agent reduces total mortality in the first 30 days after a suspected myocardial infarction by 30 percent compared with a placebo ($p < 0.002$). Which of the following questions would be the most important to have answered?

(A) Was the trial blinded?
(B) What was the power of the study?
(C) What happened to surviving patients in the next year?
(D) What percentage of patients in each group actually had a myocardial infarction?
(E) What was the effect on mortality from coronary heart disease?

54. A radiologist develops a new screening test for cancer of the pancreas. The sensitivity and specificity of the test are said to be "very high, at least 98 percent." You are asked to determine whether it would be useful to screen everyone in your primary care practice with this test in the next year. To answer, you would need to know all the following EXCEPT

(A) the incidence of asymptomatic pancreatic cancer
(B) the prevalence of asymptomatic pancreatic cancer
(C) the exact values of the sensitivity and specificity of the tests
(D) the cost of the test
(E) the survival rate from pancreatic cancer cases detected by the new test

Questions 55–57

In a study of the effectiveness of pertussis vaccine in preventing pertussis (whooping cough), the following data were collected by studying siblings of children who had the disease.

Immunization Status of Sibling Contact	Number of Siblings Exposed to Case	Number of Cases among Siblings
Complete	4,000	400
None	1,000	400

55. What was the secondary attack rate of pertussis in fully immunized household contacts?

(A) 0 percent
(B) 10 percent
(C) 25 percent
(D) 40 percent
(E) 75 percent

56. What was the protective efficacy of whooping cough vaccine?

(A) 25 percent
(B) 40 percent
(C) 75 percent
(D) 90 percent
(E) None of the above

57. What was the relative risk of contacting whooping cough in the unimmunized children compared with the fully immunized children?

(A) 0.25
(B) 0.5
(C) 1.0
(D) 2.0
(E) 4.0

Questions 58–63

Data from an investigation of an epidemic of German measles in a remote village in Brazil are given in the table below:

Age Group (years)	Number in Population	Number Ill (symptomatic)	Number Not Ill but with Antibody Rise (asymptomatic)	Number Uninfected	Percent Infected
0–9	204	110	74	20	90
10–19	129	70	46	13	90
20–39	161	88	57	16	90
40–59	78	42	28	8	90
60+	42	2	2	38	10
Totals	614	312	207	95	

58. Which expression represents the calculation to determine the incidence of illness for all age groups (as a percentage)?

(A) $\dfrac{312}{614} \times 100\% = 50.8\%$

(B) $\dfrac{207}{614} \times 100\% = 33.7\%$

(C) $\dfrac{95}{519} \times 100\% = 18.3\%$

(D) $\dfrac{519}{614} \times 100\% = 84.5\%$

(E) $\dfrac{207}{519} \times 100\% = 39.9\%$

59. Which expression represents the calculation to determine the percentage of infection that is asymptomatic (subclinical)?

(A) $\dfrac{312}{614} \times 100\% = 50.8\%$

(B) $\dfrac{207}{614} \times 100\% = 33.7\%$

(C) $\dfrac{95}{519} \times 100\% = 18.3\%$

(D) $\dfrac{519}{614} \times 100\% = 84.5\%$

(E) $\dfrac{207}{519} \times 100\% = 39.9\%$

60. Based on the age specific infection rates, when did German measles previously occur in this village—in relation to the current epidemic?

(A) 1 to 9 years ago
(B) 10 to 19 years ago
(C) 20 to 39 years ago
(D) 40 to 59 years ago
(E) 60 years ago

61. The authors of a study state that careful autopsies show that 60 percent of all persons who die have evidence of recent or previous pulmonary embolism and conclude that pulmonary embolism is the leading cause of death in the U.S. Possible reasons for disagreeing with the conclusion include all the following EXCEPT

(A) confounding
(B) selection bias
(C) random error
(D) lack of definition of pulmonary embolism
(E) lead-time bias

62. "The absence of valvular calcification in an adult suggests that severe valvular aortic stenosis is not present." This statement means that

(A) valvular calcification is a sensitive test for severe valvular aortic stenosis
(B) valvular calcification is an insensitive test for severe valvular aortic stenosis
(C) valvular calcification is a specific test for severe valvular aortic stenosis
(D) valvular calcification is a nonspecific test for severe valvular aortic stenosis
(E) the positive predictive value of valvular calcification is high

63. Current techniques for estimating the number of cancers caused by low-level radiation are based primarily on

(A) data from women who have undergone mammography
(B) data from atomic bomb victims
(C) the Ames model
(D) cohort studies of x-ray technicians
(E) none of the above

64. In a previously well 35-year-old man with 3 h of severe, crushing substernal chest pain and 5 mm of acute ST elevation in leads V_2 to V_4, application of Bayesian reasoning would indicate that

(A) he is likely to have a nonatherosclerotic form of coronary heart disease
(B) he is likely to have a serum cholesterol above 9 mmol/L (326 mg/dL)
(C) he is likely to be having an acute myocardial infarction
(D) an elevated level of a creatine kinase MB isozyme is likely to be a false positive
(E) measurement of creatine kinase MB isozymes would not be a very sensitive test

65. Decision analyses often include a patient's utilities in the determination of the best decision. These utilities measure

(A) whether a patient favors one decision over another
(B) whether a physician favors one decision over another
(C) the difference between a patient's decision and the physician's decision
(D) the relative value a patient places on a particular outcome
(E) the relative likelihood of a particular outcome

66. A decision analysis of the appropriate treatment of suspected herpes encephalitis shows that the decision whether to treat with acyclovir is insensitive to the likelihood of severe complications of brain biopsy needed to make the diagnosis. This implies that

(A) a brain biopsy has a low sensitivity for the diagnosis of herpes simplex encephalitis
(B) a brain biopsy has a low specificity for the diagnosis of herpes simplex encephalitis
(C) a brain biopsy has a high specificity for the diagnosis of herpes simplex encephalitis
(D) the exact frequency of severe complications following brain biopsy is not important
(E) acyclovir therapy is unlikely to be successful in a patient who has had a brain biopsy

DIRECTIONS: Each group of questions below consists of lettered headings followed by a set of numbered items. For each numbered item select the **one** lettered heading with which it is **most** closely associated. Each lettered heading may be used **once, more than once, or not at all.**

Questions 67–70

For each of the studies below, choose the most appropriate statistical test to analyze the data.

   (A) Chi-square analysis
   (B) Student t test
   (C) Analysis of variance
   (D) Paired t test
   (E) Linear regression

67. Comparison of systolic blood pressures in independent samples of pregnant and nonpregnant women

68. Comparison of the prevalence of hepatitis B surface antigen (HBsAg) in medical and dental students

69. Comparison of the level of blood glucose in male and female rats following administration of three different drugs

70. Comparison of serum cholesterol before and after ingestion of hamburgers in a sample of fast-food patrons

Questions 71–74

For each of the following descriptions, pick the appropriate epidemiologic term.

   (A) Confounding
   (B) Effect modification
      (interaction)
   (C) Misclassification bias
   (D) Lead-time bias
   (E) None of the above

71. Elevated bilirubin levels in neonates are associated with brain damage only in babies who also have infections or severe hemolytic disease

72. People who drink coffee tend to smoke more, and for this reason coffee drinkers have a higher risk of lung cancer

73. Higher lead levels in hyperactive children may be due to increased consumption of paint in children who were already hyperactive

74. The association between blood lead levels and IQ may be a result of the fact that both are associated with socioeconomic status

Questions 75–78

In each statement below, data are presented based on a cohort study of coronary heart disease. Choose the parameter that best describes each of these statements.

(A) Point prevalence
(B) Incidence rate
(C) Standardized morbidity ratio
(D) Relative risk
(E) None of the above

75. At the initial examination, 17 persons per 1,000 had evidence of coronary heart disease (CHD)

76. Among heavy smokers, the observed frequency of angina pectoris was 1.6 times as great as the expected frequency during the first 12 years of the study

77. During the first 8 years of the study, 45 persons developed coronary heart disease per 1,000 persons who entered the study free of disease

78. The risk of coronary heart disease was 23 percent higher in relatives of patients with CHD than in the general population

Questions 79–83

Match the examples below with the appropriate epidemiologic terms.

(A) Lead-time bias
(B) Surveillance bias
(C) Recall bias
(D) Type 1 error
(E) Power

79. Medical students who fail a physiology examination are more likely to report missing two or more physiology lectures than those who fail a neuroanatomy examination

80. The chance of discovering the truth that twice as many of your friends are at the movies as are studying for their board examinations

81. In a class of 150 medical students, there will likely be a few who can answer this question correctly without understanding the material

82. The likelihood of finding a lost biochemistry notebook in your apartment is higher in the month of June than in the month of March

83. Medical students enrolled in a first-year anatomy class are more likely to remain at their same addresses for the next 2 years than medical students enrolled in fourth-year clerkships

Questions 84–87

Choose the rate that best describes each statement below.

(A) Secondary attack rate
(B) Case-fatality rate
(C) Morbidity rate
(D) Age-adjusted mortality
(E) Crude mortality

84. Death occurs in 10 percent of cases of meningococcal meningitis

85. Approximately 9 people die each year in the United States for every 1,000 estimated to be alive

86. Eighty percent of susceptible household contacts of a child with chickenpox develop this disease

87. Children between the ages of 1 and 5 have an average of eight colds per year

Questions 88–91

For each of the descriptions of statistical procedures below, choose the statistical error.

(A) Observations are not independent
(B) Variable is not normally distributed
(C) Unequal group sizes or unequal variances
(D) Not enough degrees of freedom
(E) None of the above

88. The frequencies of infection of the urinary tract are compared in 24 children treated with intermittent catheterization and 9 children treated with urinary diversion. In the catheterization group, 85/231 urine cultures were positive, compared with 34/55 in the diversion group. The difference between these two proportions was statistically significant ($\chi^2 = 11.4$, degrees of freedom = 1.0, p < 0.001)

89. The mean lengths of hospital stay were compared in 20 premature infants treated surgically and 20 premature infants treated medically for patent ductus arteriosus. The mean lengths of stay in the two groups were 50 ± 30 and 30 ± 30 days (mean $\pm$ standard deviation), respectively. The t test was not significant (t = 1.5, p = 0.07)

90. The parity of 100 women with breast cancer was compared with that of 200 controls. Among the cases, 40 percent were nulliparous, 30 percent had one child, and 30 percent had more than one child; among the controls the numbers were 20, 30, and 50 percent, respectively. The mean ($\pm$ SD) parity in the cases was 1.6 ± 2.1; in the controls it was 2.2 ± 2.3. The difference was statistically significant using the t test ($t = -2.2$; $p = 0.04$)

91. An investigator wishes to examine the efficacy of varicella vaccine. For convenience, he randomizes four classes of third graders for the study: two classes receive the vaccine and two do not. Over the next year, only 2/57 children in the vaccine group, but 25/60 children in the control group get chickenpox ($\chi^2 = 23$, degrees of freedom $= 1.0$, $p < 0.001$). The investigator concludes that the vaccine is highly effective

---

Questions 92–95

For each of the studies described below, select the critical statement that best explains why the conclusion is misleading or false.

(A) Lack of a control group
(B) Lack of proper follow-up
(C) Lack of adjustment for age
(D) Lack of denominators
(E) Lack of adjustment for race

92. Of 250 consecutive, unselected women in whom acute cholecystitis was diagnosed, 75 were under age 50 and 175 were over age 50. The investigator concluded that older women are at greater risk of acute cholecystitis than are younger women

93. In a review of 3,000 patients in whom adult-onset diabetes was diagnosed, 2,000 of these patients were obese at the time of diagnosis. The investigator concluded that there was an association between diabetes and obesity

94. Acute anxiety neurosis was diagnosed among 250 patients and follow-up data were available on 80 percent of these patients 10 years later. The mortality experience of this cohort was no different than that of the general population. The authors concluded that the diagnosis of acute anxiety neurosis was not associated with a decrease in longevity

95. Of 143 patients who died of bacterial endocarditis and on whom autopsies were performed, 2 percent were less than 10 years of age. The authors concluded that bacterial endocarditis is rare in childhood

Questions 96–99

Choose the term that best fits the description.

(A) Matching
(B) Stratification
(C) Age adjustment
(D) Multivariate statistical analysis
(E) Survival analysis

96. In a cohort study of hypertensive men, the proportions of subjects with high and low renin levels who survived for 5 years are compared separately among those aged 40 to 49, those aged 50 to 59, and those aged 60 to 69 at entry

97. A sampling strategy is used to achieve comparability of the groups being studied

98. A technique that takes into account variable length of follow-up is used

99. Six different risk ratios are calculated: one for each sex at each of three social class levels

Questions 100–103

The following two-by-two table represents the findings of a 5-year cohort study in which the incidence of suicide in veterans who served in Vietnam was compared with that of veterans who served elsewhere. Match the name of the parameter below with the appropriate formula.

	Suicide	No Suicide
Served in Vietnam	a	b
Served elsewhere	c	d

(A) ad/bc
(B) $(a + b)/(a + b + c + d)$
(C) $(a + c)/(a + b + c + d)$
(D) $[a/(a + b)]/[c/(c + d)]$
(E) $a/(a + b) - c/(c + d)$

100. The odds ratio

101. The relative risk

102. The excess risk of suicide in Vietnam veterans

103. The overall incidence (per 5 years) of suicide in the study

Questions 104–107

Match each description of a sampling procedure with the correct term.

(A) Systematic sampling
(B) Paired sampling
(C) Simple random sampling
(D) Stratified sampling
(E) Cluster sampling

104. Each individual of the total group has an equal chance of being selected

105. Households are selected at random, and every person in each household is included in the sample

106. Individuals are initially assembled according to some order in a group and then individuals are selected according to some constant determinant; e.g., every fourth subject is selected

107. Individuals are divided into subgroups on the basis of specified characteristics and then random samples are selected from each subgroup

Questions 108–112

A new test for chlamydial infections of the cervix is introduced. Half of the women who are tested have a positive test. Compared with the gold standard of careful cultures, 45 percent of those with a positive test are infected with chlamydia, and 95 percent of those with a negative test are free of the infection. Match the epidemiologic terms below with the correct percentage.

(A) 5 percent
(B) 25 percent
(C) 80 percent
(D) 90 percent
(E) None of the above

108. Sensitivity of the test

109. Specificity of the test

110. Prevalence of chlamydial infection in that community

111. Predictive value of a positive test

112. Predictive value of a negative test

Questions 113–116

Select the letter corresponding to the figure that best fits each description.

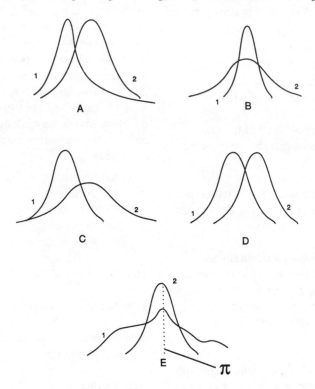

113. Distributions 1 and 2 have the same median and mean, but 2 has the greater variance

114. Distributions 1 and 2 have the same variance, but different means

115. Compared with curve 2, curve 1 is skewed to the right

116. This figure represents a tasty dessert

Questions 117-120

For each result or conclusion described below, select the choice that might best explain it.

(A) Ecologic fallacy
(B) Type 1 error
(C) Type 2 error
(D) Selection bias
(E) Misclassification bias

117. A randomized blinded trial of aspirin to prevent myocardial infarction fails to find a difference between aspirin and placebo groups after 5 years (N = 500 per group; p = 0.11)

118. A study of patterns of contraceptive use finds that counties with the highest per capita use of condoms also have the highest pregnancy rates (N = 100,000; p < 0.001) and concludes that condoms are ineffective as contraceptives

119. An investigator analyzes data from the National Health Interview Survey and finds that there is a positive association between consumption of turkey and degenerative joint disease in black women 50 to 59 years old (N = 50; p < 0.05)

120. In a case-control study of lung cancer, cases' spouses are chosen as controls. The odds ratio for smoking is 3.0, which does not quite reach statistical significance (N = 30 per group; p = 0.07)

Questions 121-125

For each variable described below, choose the type of measurement scale.

(A) Dichotomous scale
(B) Nominal scale
(C) Ordinal scale
(D) Interval scale
(E) Ratio scale

121. Survival of a particular patient for at least 5 years

122. Frequency of somnolence during biochemistry lectures: never, sometimes, usually, or always

123. Birth weight

124. Type of medical specialty

125. Year of birth

ACDBD

CA A P
B D A E

Questions 126–130

Dr. Vera Blues, a noted psychiatric epidemiologist, is interested in the diagnosis of depression. She develops a new test for its diagnosis, which she calls the Blues test. According to the gold standard, which involves meeting the *DSM III* criteria, about 1 percent of adults in the U.S. are depressed. Dr. Blues studies her new test in 100 persons diagnosed as being depressed by the gold standard; 80 have a positive Blues test. She finds 400 persons who are not depressed; again, 80 have a positive test. She reports her findings in the *Journal of the Society of Academic Psychiatrists (JSAP)*. Match the statements that Dr. Blues made in her article with the appropriate percentage.

(A) 80 percent
(B) 50 percent
(C) 20 percent
(D) < 1 percent
(E) None of the above

126. "I found that the sensitivity of the Blues test was..."

127. "The specificity of the Blues test was..."

128. "The likelihood that someone with depression would have a positive Blues test was..."

129. "The likelihood that someone in the population with a positive Blues test would be depressed was..."

130. "The likelihood that someone in the population with a negative Blues test would be depressed was..."

Biostatistics and Methods of Epidemiology

Answers

1.   The answer is D. *(Mausner, ed 2. p 1.)* The word *epidemiology* comes from the Greek words *epi* (upon) and *demos* (people). In fact, there is a separate word for the study of determinants of disease in animals—*epizootiology*. Epidemiology is the study of both the distribution of diseases in human populations and the determinants of the observed distribution. It began as the study of infectious diseases but has expanded to include the study of chronic diseases, organization of health care, delivery of health care, and occupational and environmental health.

2.   The answer is A. *(Ingelfinger, ed 2. pp 11–12.)* Two characteristics are independent of each other (i.e., unrelated) if and only if the probability of both occurring in the same person is equal to the product of their probabilities. In this example, we estimate the probability of hearing impairment in this population as $120/1,000 = 0.12$, and the probability of diabetes as $50/1,000 = 0.05$. The product of these probabilities is $(0.12)(0.05) = 0.006$. Thus, with a sample size of 1,000, if hearing impairment and diabetes were independent, we would expect about 6 persons to be both hearing-impaired and diabetic—exactly what was found.

3.   The answer is C. *(Colton, pp 31, 189–195.)* The *standard deviation* (SD) is a measure of the variability or scatter of a set of observations about the mean. A large SD means that the observations are widely scattered about the mean, whereas a small SD indicates that they are clustered closely about the mean. The *standard error of the mean* (*SEM*) is a measure of the variability of a sample mean. Thus, whereas the SD reflects scatter of observations about the (sample or population) mean, the SEM reflects scatter of sample means around the true population mean. The larger the sample, the closer its mean is likely to be to the population mean. Thus, as the sample size increases, the standard error of the mean decreases. Mathematically, the SEM is equal to the sample standard deviation divided by the square root of the sample size $(SD/\sqrt{n})$. The *range* describes the variability only in terms of the smallest and largest values without indicating the distribution of the values about the mean. The *regression* and *correlation coefficients* are measures of the degree of relationship between two variables.

4.   The answer is C. *(Mausner, ed 2. pp 156–158.)* This study is a *cohort* (prospective) study because the subjects (pregnant women) were categorized on the basis of exposure or lack of exposure to a risk factor (smoking during pregnancy), and then were followed to determine if a particular outcome (low-birth-weight babies) resulted. The term *cohort* refers to the group of subjects who are followed forward in time to see which ones develop the outcome. *Clinical trials* are prospective studies in which an *intervention* is applied—no intervention was mentioned in the question. In a *case-control* (retrospective) study of the relationship between low birth weight and maternal smoking, infants would be selected on the basis of low birth weight (cases) and normal birth weight (controls) and then the frequency of maternal smoking would be compared in the two groups. In *cross-sectional* studies exposure and outcome are measured at the same point in time.

5.   The answer is B. *(Ingelfinger, ed 2. pp 189–191.)* Although hypertension can resolve spontaneously, this is an unlikely explanation for resolution over a 2-week period in 35 percent of the subjects. A much more likely explanation is *regression toward the mean*. Because of random fluctuations, any one measurement of blood pressure may be far from a person's normal blood pressure. By referring patients for the study based on a single measurement, those in whom the measurement was falsely high are much more likely to be referred than those in whom the measurement was too low. Thus in any group selected based on a characteristic with substantial day-to-day variation, many will have values closer to the population mean when the measurement is repeated. Neither baseline drift (which occurs with measurements on certain machines requiring frequent calibration) nor measurement error is as likely an explanation. The Hawthorne effect refers to a tendency among study subjects to change simply because they are being studied. It is much more likely to affect studies of behavior or attitudes than a study of blood pressure.

6.   The answer is B. *(Colton, pp 71–73.)* The overall probability of reaching stage IV is 10 percent; i.e., of 100 patients, about 10 would be expected to reach stage IV. However, if it is given that the patient has reached stage II, that patient has missed his or her chance to stop at stage I, so the probability of reaching stage IV is a little greater. In fact, since 30 of 100 patients get no farther than stage I, only 70 make it to stage II or more. Of these, 10 will make it to stage IV. The probability of reaching stage IV given that one has reached stage II is thus about 10/70 (14 percent).

7.   The answer is D. *(Colton, pp 129, 174.)* The data presented are for a dichotomous predictor variable (book/no book) and a dichotomous outcome variable (dysfunction/no dysfunction), so a chi-square test (but not a t test) is appropriate for analysis. Since there is apparently such a big difference between the groups, chance is not a likely explanation for the findings. It is essential to know how the groups were assigned if the study is to be properly interpreted. In fact, in this case, we chose the control group from subjects at a clinic for sexual dysfunction.

8.   The answer is D. *(Mausner, ed 2. pp 46–48.)* Person-years of observation are frequently used in the denominator of incidence rates and provide a method of dealing with variable follow-up periods. Person-years of observation simultaneously take into account the number of persons under observation and the duration of observation of each person. For example, if 8 new cases of diabetes occurred among 1,000 people followed for 2 years, the incidence would be 8 cases per 2,000 person-years, or 4 per 1,000 person-years of follow-up. The distinction between *rates* and *proportions* is not well maintained in standard epidemiologic terminology. Rates should have units of inverse time and will vary depending on the units of measurement of time; they can vary from 0 to infinity. However, such terms as *case-fatality rate, attack rate,* and *prevalence rate* are in widespread usage even though technically they are all proportions; i.e., they vary between 0 and 1 and are unitless.

9.   The answer is C. *(Ingelfinger, ed 2. pp 37–46.)* The chance of remaining uninfected for 1 year is 0.7; for 3 years it is $(0.7)(0.7)(0.7) = 0.343$. Everyone who does not remain uninfected must become infected; thus the chance of becoming infected is $1 - 0.343 = 0.657$, or about 66 percent.

10.   The answer is C. *(Mausner, ed 2. pp 256–257.)* Net growth rate equals the birth rate minus the death rate plus the in-migration rate minus the out-migration rate: $(17 - 10) + 2 = 9$. Rates can be added or subtracted directly only if they are based on the same population denominator (in this case, the estimated midyear population).

11.   The answer is E. *(Colton, pp 28–31.)* The correct values for mean, median, and mode are 3.4, 3, and 2. The *mean* is the average: the sum of the observations divided by the number of observations. In this case, the mean is $31 \div 9 = 3.4$. The *median* is the middle observation in a series of ordered observations, i.e., the 50th percentile (when the number of observations is even, it is midway between the two middle observations). In this case, when the observations are ordered—1,2,2,2,3,4,4,6,7—the median is 3. The *mode* is the observation that occurs with greatest frequency; in this case it is 2, which occurs three times.

12.   The answer is D. *(Mausner, ed 2. pp 44–49.)* According to the table, 10 new cases of tuberculosis developed among the 500 persons belonging to households with a case of tuberculosis at the time of the first survey. Because these 500 persons were followed for 2 years, the number of person-years of exposure is 1,000. Therefore, the incidence rate is calculated as follows:

$$\frac{10 \text{ new cases}}{500 \text{ persons} \times 2 \text{ years}} = 10 \text{ cases per } 1,000 \text{ person-years}$$

(See also question 8.)

13. The answer is C. *(Mausner, ed 2. pp 44–49.)* Ten new cases of tuberculosis developed among 10,000 persons belonging to households that had no culture-positive cases at the time of the first survey. Since these 10,000 persons were followed for 2 years, the number of person-years of exposure is 20,000. Therefore, the incidence rate is calculated as follows:

$$\frac{10 \text{ new cases}}{10,000 \text{ persons} \times 2 \text{ years}} = 0.5 \text{ cases per 1,000 person-years}$$

14. The answer is E. *(Mausner, ed 2. p 169.)* The relative risk is the *ratio* of the incidence of a disease in a group exposed to a factor (in this case, household contact with tuberculosis) to the incidence in a group not exposed to the factor (persons without household contact). Therefore, the relative risk is

$$\frac{\text{Incidence in households with exposure}}{\text{Incidence in households without exposure}} = \frac{10}{0.5} = 20$$

Identification of groups with a high level of relative risk can be useful in planning disease control programs.

15. The answer is D. *(Mausner, ed 2. pp 289–292.)* The identification of a specific factor (food) as a cause of illness (food poisoning) depends on comparing the proportion who became ill among those who did and those who did not eat each specified food (the proportion ill is sometimes called the "attack rate," but in fact it is a proportion, not a rate [see question 8]). The proportion ill among those who ate the food suspected of causing the disease should be significantly greater than among those who did not eat the food.

16. The answer is C. *(Colton, pp 115–119.)* The null hypothesis generally is that there is no difference between groups. The p value is the probability of obtaining a difference between groups at least as great as that observed in the study *if the null hypothesis were true*. Because it is calculated under the *assumption* that the null hypothesis is true, it cannot actually estimate the probability of the null hypothesis. The investigator and readers of the study, in interpreting the results, must decide whether the p value is low enough to warrant rejection of the null hypothesis. The value of p below which the null hypothesis will be rejected (most often 0.05) is known as "alpha." If the p value is greater than alpha, the results are regarded as not statistically significant and the null hypothesis is not rejected. This, of course, does not mean that the two groups really are equivalent, only that the data did not provide sufficient evidence to conclude that they are different.

17. The answer is E. *(Mausner, ed 2. pp 155–156.)* In *experimental* studies, the investigators determine exposure of the study and control groups to a suspected causal factor and measure responses in the two groups. In *observational* studies, investigators have no control over exposure to a suspected causal factor but can measure responses in those who are and are not exposed. In both types of studies, the attempt is made to use study and control groups similar in regard to all variables except exposure to the factor under study.

18. The answer is E. *(Schlesselman, pp 135-138.)* Misclassification bias—i.e., including people who do not really have the disease (controls) in the case groups—will tend to make the odds ratio falsely close to 1, rather than falsely high. (In the extreme example where misclassification is so bad that both case and control groups are really equal mixtures of cases and controls, the odds ratio necessarily would equal 1.) Recall bias could cause a falsely high odds ratio; it is potentially a problem when using maternal recall to investigate exposures associated with birth defects. It is less likely to be a problem for an exposure such as smoking than for an exposure that controls are more likely to forget. This study *is* a case-control study: the risk factor in this case is prenatal exposure to cigarette smoke. The placebo effect is of concern in unblinded intervention studies; it refers to the tendency of subjects to report improvement even when the treatment is not effective. It has no relevance to case-control studies.

19. The answer is B. *(Colton, pp 125-127.)* Since undescended testes are uncommon, the odds ratio in this study approximates the relative risk (risk ratio). The fact that the 95 percent confidence interval excludes 1.0 means that $p < 0.05$. Confidence intervals describe the range of values not significantly different from the observed value, with a type 1 error rate (alpha) of 1.0 minus the level of confidence. Thus, a 95 percent confidence interval shows the numbers that are not significantly different statistically from what was observed at the 5 percent level. The lower the level of confidence, the narrower the confidence interval, so a 90 percent confidence interval would be narrower than a 95 percent confidence interval, in this case excluding 1.0 for certain. Thus, if the study is accurate, it suggests that baby boys whose mothers smoke are 2.6 times as likely to have undescended testes.

20. The answer is D. *(Colton, pp 63-70.)* For two events or conditions, the probability that either will occur is the sum of their probabilities, minus the probability that both will occur. This is illustrated in the following figure:

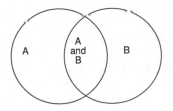

If we simply add the probability of A to the probability of B, the area labeled "A and B" will get counted twice. Therefore, the probability of (A and B) must be subtracted from the sum of the probabilities: $p(A \text{ or } B) = p(A) + p(B) - p(A \text{ and } B)$. In this question, it is specifically stated that the two conditions are independent. When that is the case, the probability that both will occur is the product of their probabilities: $p(A \text{ and } B) = p(A) \times p(B)$. The answer to this problem is $0.1 + 0.5 - (0.1)(0.5) = 0.55$. Note that another common situation is when two conditions are mutually exclusive rather than independent (i.e., the probability that both will occur is zero). In this case, the probability of either one's occurring is simply the sum of their probabilities. For example, if condition A were blue eyes and condition B brown eyes, the probability of either blue or brown eyes would be 0.60.

21. The answer is D. *(Sackett, pp 127–131.)* Decision analysis begins with construction of a decision tree, i.e., outlining all possible outcomes, good and bad, of each decision. The next step involves estimation of the probabilities of these outcomes under each possible decision. The outcomes are then given ratings called *utilities*, which correspond to their relative desirability. The utilities and probabilities are then used together to compute the expected value of different decisions. Finally, in a process called *sensitivity analysis*, the probabilities and utilities are varied to see how this affects the expected values of the different decisions. Calculation of sample size is not necessary for decision analysis because decision analysis is basically a pencil-and-paper (and computer) exercise; it does not require study subjects.

22. The answer is B. *(Colton, pp 189–190.)* Because the goal of the study is to determine the correlation between serum levels of sodium and antidiuretic hormone (ADH) in patients who have meningitis, simultaneous determination of these paired variables in each member of a group of patients should be performed. The design described in choice A will allow only determination of the correlation within an individual or the variability of the assay methods; the design described in choice C will allow determination of the mean values of each variable but not their relationship; and the design described in choice D will permit comparison of ADH in cases and controls but will not provide data on serum levels of sodium.

23. The answer is D. *(Ingelfinger, ed 2. pp 91–95.)* The normal (Gaussian) distribution is a symmetric, bell-shaped distribution with many useful mathematical properties. Because it is symmetric and unimodal, the mean is equal to the median and mode. It is entirely described by just two parameters: the mean and the standard deviation. The mean determines the location of the curve, the standard deviation how flat it is. As values get farther and farther from the mean, they become increasingly unlikely. Thus there are many more observations between 0 and 1 standard deviation from the mean than there are between 1 and 2 standard deviations from the mean. Approximately 68 percent of observations fall within 1 standard deviation of the mean, 95 percent within 2 standard deviations, and 99.7 percent within 3 standard deviations.

24.   The answer is B. *(Ingelfinger, ed 2. p 723.)* Sensitivity and specificity are measures of how often a diagnostic test gives the correct answer. Sensitivity reflects the test's performance in people who *have* the disease, and specificity measures the test's performance in people who *do not have* the disease. These definitions can be illustrated as follows:

	Disease Present	Disease Absent
Test Positive	True Positive (TP)	False Positive (FP)
Test Negative	False Negative (FN)	True Negative (TN)

Sensitivity = TP / (TP + FN)   Specificity = TN / (TN + FP)

Among people who have the disease, there are two possibilities: either the test correctly identifies them (TP), or it falsely classifies them as negative (FN). Thus among those with disease, sensitivity measures how often the test gives the right answer. (A good way to remember sensitivity is by the initials PID: positive in disease.) Similarly, among people who do not have the disease, there are also two possibilities: either the test will correctly identify them as not having disease (TN), or it will falsely classify them as diseased (FP). Thus specificity measures how often the test gives the right answer among those who do not have the disease. (A good way to remember specificity is by the initials NIH: negative in health.)

As opposed to sensitivity and specificity, which measure the test's performance in groups of patients who do and do not have the disease, *predictive value* measures how often the test is right in patients grouped another way: by whether the test result is positive or negative. Thus, predictive value of a positive test is the proportion of positive tests that are true positives [TP / (TP + FP)], and predictive value of a negative result is the proportion of negative test results that are true negatives [TN / (TN + FN)].

But predictive value is a little tricky because it also depends on the *prevalence* of the disease in the population tested. In this case, Dr. Stewells assembled groups of 100 patients with and without cholera, and the prevalence is not given. Therefore, predictive value cannot be calculated in this question, and the correct answer is B, since specificity is 88 percent, not 12 percent.

25.   The answer is C. *(Ingelfinger, ed 2 pp 7 23.)* In this study of 1,000 patients with profuse diarrhea, 343 of them had cholera. Thus the prevalence of cholera (in this population) was 343/1,000. (Note that this is not an incidence because we are measuring existing cases, rather than new cases occurring over a period of time.) The predictive value of a positive result can thus be directly determined as TP/(TP + FP) = 312/(312 + 79) = 80 percent. Similarly, the predictive value of a negative result is TN/(TN + FN) = 578/(578 + 31) = 95 percent. Note here that this predictive value refers to the predictive value of the test in patients *admitted to the hospital with profuse diarrhea*. Since prevalence data from the general population are still lacking, the usefulness of this test in the general population is undefined. Predictably, the positive predictive value of this test in an asymptomatic population will be less.

26.   The answer is B. *(Ingelfinger, ed 2. pp 7–23.)* As the prevalence falls, more and more of those tested will *not* have cholera. This would change neither the sensitivity nor specificity of the test, which do not depend on disease prevalence, but would affect predictive value: as prevalence falls, predictive value of a positive result also falls, whereas predictive value of a negative result rises. This makes sense: As a disease becomes more and more unlikely, positive test results should be viewed with increasing skepticism, whereas negative results become increasingly believable.

27.   The answer is A. *(Colton, p 257.)* Randomization is the use of a predetermined plan of allocation or assignment of subjects to treatment groups such that assignment occurs solely by chance. It is used to eliminate bias on the part of the investigator and the subject in the choice of treatment group. The goal of randomization is to allow chance to distribute unknown sources of biologic variability equally to the treatment and control groups. However, because chance does determine assignment, significant differences between the groups may arise, especially if the number of subjects is small. Therefore, whenever randomization is used, the comparability of the treatment groups should be assessed to determine whether or not balance was achieved.

28.   The answer is D. *(Colton, pp 115–117.)* A p value of 0.60 indicates that the observed (or a greater) difference between the means could occur by chance as often as 6 times out of 10. This is not the same as saying that this result did occur by chance. Such a probability of chance is usually interpreted to mean that the result is not statistically significant. A value of p of 0.05 is the conventional upper limit of significance. However, even though $p = 0.60$, the null hypothesis of no difference between the means is not proved to be true. The most that can be said when the p value is not statistically significant is that the data are insufficient to cast doubt on the truth of the null hypothesis. If the samples were larger in size, the difference might be found to be statistically significant.

29.   The answer is B. *(Mausner, ed 2. pp 156–159.)* The study described was a case-control study. In this type of study, people who have a disease (cases) are compared with people whom they closely resemble except for the presence of the disease under study (controls). Cases and controls are then studied for the frequency of exposure to a suspected risk factor. In case-control studies, the validity of inferences about the causal relationship between the exposure (cigarette smoking) and the disease (lung cancer) depends on how comparable the cases and controls are for all variables that may be related to both the risk factor and disease under study (e.g., age, sex, race, place of residence, and occupation).

30.   The answer is D. *(Last, ed 2. p 9.)* Because circumcised males are at lower risk of UTI, urine cultures will have a lower yield in that group. In uncircumcised boys, the proportion of UTIs attributable to lack of circumcision is (RR−1)/RR. Since RR = 10, 90 percent of UTIs in uncircumcised males appear to be due to the fact that those males are uncircumcised. Therefore, imaging their urinary tracts in hopes of finding another predisposing factor for UTI is likely to have a much *lower* yield than similar imaging in a circumcised boy.

31–33.   The answers are: 31–D, 32–B, 33–E. *(Rothman, pp 311–313.)* The *excess risk* is the incidence in those exposed to the risk factors minus the incidence in those unexposed. Thus, the excess risk from drinking among nonsmokers is 30 − 10 = 20 cases per 10,000 person-years. Similarly, for smoking (among nondrinkers) it is 50 − 10 = 40 cases per 10,000 person-years. The *relative risk* for smoking among nondrinkers is 50/10 = 5.0, but the overall relative risk also depends on the relative risk in drinkers, which may be higher, lower, or the same. The overall relative risk also depends on the proportion of the population that drinks: the lower that proportion, the closer the overall relative risk will be to that of nondrinkers. To determine which risk factor is the cause of a greater number of cases (*population attributable fraction*, sometimes called *attributable risk*) requires knowledge of the prevalence of the risk factor, as well as its relative risk.

When there is more than one risk factor for a disease, it is important to compare the risk in those with both risk factors with that expected under different models of causation. Under an additive model, when risk factors are independent, *excess risks add*. Thus the excess risk for smoking and drinking would be 20 + 40 = 60. To give an excess risk of 60 requires that X = 70.

Under a multiplicative model, when risk factors are independent, *relative risks multiply*. Thus the relative risk for patients with both risk factors should be 3 × 5 = 15. Thus X must be 15 × 10 = 150.

These questions demonstrate that determining the presence of independence, synergy, or antagonism among risk factors requires clear specification of whether one is dealing with an additive or multiplicative model of causation.

34.   The answer is D. *(Mausner, ed 2. pp 43–45.)* Neither incidence nor prevalence rates of leukemia can be determined from the data given in the table without knowledge of the population at risk for leukemia and served by the study hospital. The data given provide numerators, but the lack of age-specific data on population prevents calculation of rates. The only conclusion (among those given in the question) that can be based on the data is that in the period 1970 to 1984 the number of children admitted to the hospital with a diagnosis of leukemia increased for the children 9 years old and under.

35.   The answer is C. *(Hulley, pp 212–213.)* The idea of a randomized study is to compare groups of patients who get one drug with groups of patients who get another (or placebo). Such a comparison is called a *between-groups* comparison because one whole group is compared with another. The analysis described in this question illustrates a *within-group* analysis. Within-group analyses in randomized studies are often interesting but cannot provide convincing evidence of causality. Only comparisons between entire randomized groups take advantage of the randomization to provide strong evidence for causality. In fact, the difference in mortality between those who did and did not adhere to placebo was even greater: 15 percent versus 28 percent. Thus, something related to taking study medication (active or not) appears to have been a strong predictor of mortality.

36. The answer is C. *(Lilienfeld, ed 2. pp 217-218.)* The attributable risk estimates the importance of a particular risk factor as a cause of the disease. The importance depends on the prevalence of the risk factor because if hardly anyone in the population has the risk factor, it is unlikely to explain very many cases of the disease. The importance of a risk factor also depends on how strong a risk factor it is, as measured by the relative risk. The formula for calculating attributable risk is

$$\frac{p(RR - 1)}{p(RR - 1) + 1}$$

where p is the prevalence of the risk factor in the population, and RR is the relative risk of the disease for the risk factor. For smoking, p is about 0.3, and RR about 20, giving an attributable risk of about 85 percent. Note that the term *attributable risk* is defined differently by different authors, so that it is helpful to specify exactly what is meant when the term is used. Synonyms for the definition supplied here are *population attributable fraction* and *etiologic fraction*.

37. The answer is B. *(Ingelfinger, ed 2. pp 258-263.)* As a general rule, it is much easier to get a falsely negative result on a randomized blinded trial than a falsely positive result. The reason is that errors will tend to affect both treatment groups, making it harder to show a difference between them. Thus, in this question, inclusion of subjects without the ear effusion (who could not benefit from the intervention) and incorrect determination of which effusions resolved would both lead to falsely negative, not falsely positive results. Similarly, a small sample size is a reason for a falsely negative, but not a falsely positive result. Only chance (random error) or a breakdown in the blinding or randomization process would be causes of a falsely positive result.

38. The answer is B. *(Colton, pp 100-107, 115-116, 124.)* The p value depends not only on the magnitude of the difference between groups (larger differences leading to smaller p values), but also on the sample size of the study. For a true difference of a given size, the p value can be made as small as desired by increasing the sample size. However, if there really is no difference between the groups (i.e., if the null hypothesis is true), the chance of obtaining statistical significance at the

0.05 level will always be 0.05, regardless of the size of the sample. The standard error of the mean (SEM) is sometimes confused with the standard deviation (SD). Whereas the SD is a measure of dispersion of individual measurements about the mean, the SEM is a measure of variation of sample means about the population mean (see question 3). The "tails" in a significance test refer to the tails of the statistical distributions used to calculate the p values. A one-tailed test is the less conservative; i.e., it *more* often leads to rejection of the null hypothesis when it is true. Just remember: If you double the number of tails, you double the p value.

39.   The answer is C. *(Mausner, ed 2. pp 200, 348–352.)* Sample size for a clinical trial depends on the frequency with which the outcome occurs in the control group, the magnitude of the effect that is to be detected, and the type 1 and type 2 error rates, alpha and beta. (A type 1 error occurs when the study erroneously finds a difference between two groups; a type 2 error is when the two groups really are different, but the study does not reach that conclusion.) An additional consideration in prospective studies, particularly those of long duration, is loss of follow-up, including mortality from causes not under investigation. The number of subjects required for the study is not affected by the prevalence of smoking because only smokers will be enrolled.

40–41.   The answers are: 40–B, 41–C. *(Wilson, ed 12. pp 7–8.)* ROC curves are a way of graphically representing how well diagnostic tests perform. A perfect test will have a curve that rises straight up to the upper left corner, indicating 100 percent sensitivity and 100 percent specificity. A completely useless test will run along the diagonal. (The diagonal represents the line sensitivity = 1 − specificity. Any time sensitivity and specificity sum to 1.0, the test provides no information.) The points along the curve represent the tradeoff between sensitivity and specificity when the cutoff or threshold for calling the test positive is changed. As an example, point A might represent a 2.5-mm ST-segment depression as a test for coronary artery disease, whereas point B might represent 1.5 mm. If we define 2.5 mm as abnormal (point A), we will miss some cases (lower sensitivity), but have fewer false positives (higher specificity). If we want higher sensitivity, we can say anyone with ST depression of more than 1.5 mm has CAD (point B), but this is at the expense of more false positive results (lower specificity).

42.   The answer is A. *(Ingelfinger, ed 2. pp 190–197.)* The finding of a statistically significant association on linear regression analysis does not prove that an association is linear, nor that it is causal, nor that it is large or important. Exponential, logarithmic, quadratic, threshold, and many other associations can lead to statistically significant linear regression coefficients. Choice C is incorrect because it implies causality, which was not demonstrated. To be able to say that lead and IQ are *independently* associated requires knowledge that other potentially confounding variables (e.g., social class) were controlled for, as with multiple linear regression.

43. The answer is C. *(Wilson, ed 12. p 1289.)* The prevalence of ankylosing spondylitis cannot be determined from the information provided. However, a simple two-by-two table can be used to estimate the odds ratio for the association between ankylosing spondylitis and HLA-B27.

	Ankylosing Spondylitis	
	Present	Absent
HLA-B27 present	0.9	0.1
HLA-B27 absent	0.07	0.93

The odds ratio would be $(0.9 \times 0.93) \div (0.1 \times 0.07) = 119$. Because the disease (ankylosing spondylitis) is rare, the odds ratio estimates the relative risk (or relative prevalence, in this case).

44. The answer is D. *(Wilson, ed 12. p 16.)* Average life expectancy in the U.S. is about 75 years. This number should be understood as simply a projection of how long a child born today can expect to live, on average, assuming no changes in mortality during his or her lifetime. *Average* (or *mean*) life expectancy is lower than the *median* age at death, because infant mortality and deaths early in life have a profound effect in shortening average life expectancy. A 65-year-old woman has already "avoided" dying from these causes and thus would be expected to live well beyond age 75.

45. The answer is E. *(Mausner, ed 2. pp 155, 312–316.)* In cohort studies, a group of subjects is defined on the basis of certain baseline characteristics and followed over time for the development of the disease (or other outcome) under study. The incidence of disease in subjects with various characteristics can then be compared with the incidence in subjects without those characteristics. If a suitable cohort can be identified from past records, a *retrospective* cohort study is possible. Cohort studies are not necessary to estimate prevalence. The prevalence of disease is the proportion of the population who have it at one point in time. Prevalence can be estimated from cross-sectional studies.

46. The answer is B. *(Hulley, pp 75–76.)* Because the association between the risk factor (smokeless tobacco use) and the disease (oral lesions) is measured at a single point in time in a whole group of subjects, this is a *cross-sectional* study. A *case-control* study might be performed over a similar time period, but the sampling would be different: one sample would be selected from among those baseball players found to have oral lesions (the cases) and a separate sample would be selected from among those players whose mouths were normal (the controls). In a *cohort* study, the habits of a group of players initially free of the disease would be measured, and these players would be followed over time to see how many develop the lesions. A *clinical trial* involves allocation of the subjects by the investigator (usually randomly) to one of two or more treatment groups.

47. The answer is E. *(Last, ed 2. pp 63, 103.)* This is a cross-sectional study. Cross-sectional studies allow one to estimate the *prevalence* (the number of existing cases at one point in time divided by the population at risk) but not *incidence* rate (number of new cases occurring over a period of time divided by the population at risk and the period of time at risk). The *prevalence* of mouth lesions is 80/110 (73 percent) in the smokeless tobacco users.

48. The answer is B. *(Last, ed 2. pp 91-92.)* The odds ratio in this question is correct and likely to be highly statistically significant. Because the data are for two dichotomous variables, and the expected value in each cell of the table is at least 5, the chi-square test could be used to determine the statistical significance of the data. However, *when the disease is common* (as is the case in this study), *the odds ratio is very different from the risk ratio.* Thus, while the odds ratio is 45.3, the risk ratio (actually, the prevalence ratio) is (80/110)/(2/36) = 13.1. Thus, smokeless tobacco users are 13.1 not 45.3 times as likely as nonusers to have mouth lesions. Misinterpretation of the odds ratio as a risk ratio when the disease is common is one of the most frequent statistical errors in the medical literature.

49. The answer is D. *(Last, ed 2. p 9.)* Among those who have the risk factor, the proportion of those with the disease that can be explained by the risk factor is called the *attributable fraction* in the exposed. This statistic can be used clinically (as in this case) and the formula is easily memorized: (RR − 1)/RR. Recall that the relative risk of mouth lesions in smokeless tobacco users was 13.1. Thus, the proportion of mouth lesions in smokeless tobacco users attributable to smokeless tobacco is 12.1/13.1, or about 92 percent.

The answer to this problem can also be calculated without knowing the simple formula above. The prevalence of mouth lesions in the smokeless tobacco users is 80/110, or about 73 percent. The prevalence in the nonusers is 2/36, or about 6 percent. Thus, in 1,000 smokeless tobacco users, we would expect a total of 73 with mouth lesions, but 6 would have had them anyway. The proportion of the 73 that is due to smokeless tobacco use is thus (73 − 6)/73, or about 92 percent.

50. The answer is D. *(Inglefinger, ed 2. pp 8-9.)* The choice of an optimal cutoff for a screening test often involves weighing the relative benefits of sensitivity and specificity. There is no set rule about which is the more important; rather, the decision must depend upon the consequences of false positive or false negative results. For example, because there is no good treatment for amyotrophic lateral sclerosis, a delay in diagnosis (or a missed diagnosis) caused by an insensitive test would be of little consequence. But since the diagnosis of ALS could end the search for a treatable cause of the patient's symptoms, a false positive result could be devastating. Thus for ALS, specificity is far more important than sensitivity. The situation is reversed for neonatal hypothyroidism, in which consequences of a false negative test (i.e., a child with hypothyroidism is missed by the test) are much worse than consequences of a false positive test (additional tests or even unnecessary thyroid hormone).

51. The answer is B. *(Benenson, ed 15. pp 499, 509.)* An *epidemic* is the occurrence of an illness, in a specific geographic area, that clearly exceeds the normal, expected incidence. *Hyperendemic* indicates a situation in which there is a persistent transmission of a disease among most of a population (as with malaria in certain parts of Africa). *Endemic* indicates the constant presence of a disease in a specific geographic area. *Enzootic* refers to the constant presence of a disease in animals in a specific geographic area. *Pandemic* refers to the worldwide spread of an epidemic disease.

52. The answer is B. *(Benenson, ed 15. pp 497, 501.)* The incubation period is the duration of time between exposure to an infectious agent and the appearance of the first manifestation of the disease. In contrast, the decubation period is the time from the disappearance of symptoms until recovery and the absence of infectious organisms. The communicable period designates the time when the infected person can transmit the infectious agent to another person.

53. The answer is C. *(Wilson, ed 12. pp 954–956.)* The importance of blinding, while it usually cannot be overemphasized, is not relevant in a study with total mortality as the end point: it is not possible to misclassify someone as alive when that person is really dead (except with fraudulent results). Power is not relevant in a study that shows a significant effect. In a randomized study, the percentages of patients who actually had myocardial infarctions should be similar in the two groups. Total mortality is a much more important end point than mortality from coronary heart disease, but long-term follow-up is absolutely essential in determining whether a therapy is useful. Perhaps the new agent simply postpones mortality by a few days or weeks.

54. The answer is A. *(Wilson, ed 12. p 1289.)* When considering whether to screen for a disease, the prevalence rather than the incidence of asymptomatic cases is relevant, since you will be interested in knowing what proportion of your patients have the disease at the time that you institute the screening policy. (The incidence would be relevant in determining how frequently to repeat the screening test.) The exact value of the specificity in particular is extremely important; a specificity of 98 percent would have a false positive rate of 2 percent, which is 20 times higher than if the specificity is 99.9 percent. No matter how inexpensive the test is, unless the survival rate of screened patients is substantially better than the survival rate for unscreened patients, the test will not be worthwhile (this could only be established with a randomized controlled trial).

55.   The answer is B. *(Benenson, ed 15. p 501.)* The secondary attack rate of a disease is the ratio of the number of cases of a specified disease among persons exposed to index cases divided by the total number so exposed. According to the data, 400 cases of pertussis occurred among 4,000 fully immunized children who were exposed to a sibling who had the disease. The secondary attack rate, as a percentage, among fully immunized children after household exposure is, therefore,

$$\frac{400}{4,000} \times 100\% = 10\%$$

56.   The answer is C. *(Greaves, Pediatr Infect Dis 2:284–286, 1983.)* The efficacy of vaccine, or the percentage reduction in the incidence of disease in vaccinated compared with unvaccinated subjects, is given by the expression

$$\text{Protection} = \frac{\text{incidence in unvaccinated} - \text{incidence in vaccinated}}{\text{incidence in unvaccinated}} \times 100$$

$$= \frac{(400/1,000) - (400/4,000)}{400/1,000} \times 100\% = 75\%$$

57.   The answer is E. *(Last, ed 12. p 48.)* The relative risk is the ratio of the incidence rates of two groups who differ by some factor—in this instance, immunization status. The relative risk is the ratio

$$\frac{\text{Incidence rate among unimmunized children}}{\text{Incidence rate among fully immunized children}}$$

or

$$\frac{400 \text{ cases}/1,000 \text{ exposed children}}{400 \text{ cases}/4,000 \text{ exposed children}} = \frac{0.4}{0.1} = 4$$

58.   The answer is A. *(Benenson, ed 15. p 501.)* The incidence of illness (as a percentage) is the total number of persons who have symptomatic illness divided by the total population at risk, and the calculation is $(312 \div 614) \times 100\% = 50.8\%$.

59.   The answer is E. *(Benenson, ed 15. p 501.)* The percentage of cases of German measles that were asymptomatic, or subclinical, is calculated by dividing the number of asymptomatic persons by the total number of infected persons. The calculation is $[207 \div (207 + 312)] \times 100\% = 39.9\%$.

60.   The answer is E. *(Benenson, ed 15. p 501.)* Age-specific infection rates were 90 percent in all age groups 0 to 59 years of age, while the rate was 10 percent in persons over 60 years of age. The low attack rate in persons over 60 suggests that this age group had developed immunity to German measles as a result of prior exposure at least 60 years before—since there was uniform susceptibility in persons under 60.

61. The answer is E. *(Wilson, ed 12. p 1090.)* The exact proportion of deaths due to pulmonary embolism is not known and could only be determined by a study of a random sample of all persons who died. This would avoid the problem of selection bias (only certain persons undergo autopsies). The study should be large enough to avoid random error (perhaps the cited study found emboli in three of five autopsies), and the investigators should have careful and precise definitions of pulmonary embolism to avoid overdiagnosis of the condition. The association between pulmonary embolism and death may be due to confounding if some other factor causes both. Thus, pulmonary embolism, though present, may not be the cause of death. Lead-time bias refers to an apparent increase in survival among persons whose disease is detected by screening. For example, 5-year survival of cancer patients identified on screening might appear to be prolonged simply as a result of starting to count the survival time earlier in the course of disease.

62. The answer is A. *(Wilson, ed 12. p 947.)* (Notice that in this example, epidemiologic "jargon" is easier to understand than English!) A sensitive test is one that is positive in most patients with a disease. If the absence of a characteristic rules out a disease, then the test is sensitive; hardly anyone with the disease has a negative test. It is not possible to determine the specificity of this test, however, without knowing the proportion of patients *without* severe aortic stenosis who have calcification.

63. The answer is B. *(Rosenstock, p 183.)* The exact risks from low-level radiation, such as that received from mammography, are unknown and must be estimated from available data on higher levels of exposure. Atomic bomb victims have an increased risk of leukemia, breast cancer, and thyroid cancer. The rates of these diseases have been correlated with approximate radiation dose from the blast. The Ames model is not used to study the effects of radiation; it is used to test the carcinogenicity of chemical substances (those that cause mutations in bacteria may cause malignant transformations in mammalian cells).

64. The answer is C. *(Wilson, ed 12. pp 953, 992.)* Do not let the magic words "Bayesian reasoning" fool you—even a young man with this clinical history is likely to be having a myocardial infarction (MI). The vast majority of MIs, even in 35-year-old men, are due to atherosclerosis. While an elevated cholesterol would increase someone's risk of an MI, most patients with an MI will not have such a high cholesterol level; many will even have normal cholesterol levels. All the usual diagnostic tests, including measurement of creatine kinase MB isozymes, would be useful.

65.   The answer is D. *(Wilson, ed 12. pp 5-11.)* In decision analysis, utilities refer to the relative values placed on various outcomes. For example, perfect health might be assigned a utility of 100, and death assigned one of 0. What, then, would the utility be for life with moderate back pain? With careful questioning, one finds that most patients place a higher value on life with disability than would be anticipated.

66.   The answer is D. *(Wilson, ed 12. pp 5-11.)* When used in the context of a decision analysis, the phrase "the decision is insensitive to X" indicates that the exact value of X is not important. It means that the person doing the decision analysis has used a range of reasonable values for X and found that the decision is not changed by any value of X within that range. The process of checking different values of X is called a *sensitivity analysis*; if the exact value of X mattered a great deal, the analyst would say that "the decision is sensitive to the value of X."

67-70.   The answers are: 67-B, 68-A, 69-C, 70-D. *(Colton, pp 40-41, 131-133, 137-139, 174-177.)* Use of the student t test to assess the difference between the mean systolic pressures of pregnant and nonpregnant women would be appropriate since the two groups are independent samples and the outcome variable is quantitative and approximately normally distributed.

In the study comparing the occurrence of hepatitis B surface antigen in medical and dental students, use of chi-square analysis would be appropriate because both the predictor and outcome variables are dichotomous; that is, students are classified by the presence or absence of the antigen and by medical or dental student status.

To compare the levels of blood glucose in rats to whom a drug was administered, analysis of variance would be appropriate because six different groups are to be analyzed (two sexes and three drugs). Analysis of variance will permit evaluation of the effects and interaction of sex and drug on the glucose level.

The paired t test is appropriate for comparing paired (e.g., before and after) measurements. Use of the regular (student two-sample) t test in this instance is inappropriate because the two samples are not independent—the same subjects are in each.

71-74.   The answers are: 71-B, 72-A, 73-E, 74-A. *(Hulley, pp 100-103. Sackett, p 147.)* Effect modification (also called "interaction") occurs when one factor modifies the effect of another on outcome. As an example, a high bilirubin seems to be a much stronger risk factor for bilirubin-induced brain damage if the baby is sick in other ways.

Confounding occurs when the association between two variables is distorted by the fact that both are associated with a third. For example, the association between coffee and lung cancer is distorted by smoking: among nonsmokers and smokers considered separately, coffee and lung cancer may be completely unrelated, but when the two groups are combined, an association appears to be present. Similarly lead levels need to be related to IQ separately at each level of socioeconomic status to assure that the association is not due to confounding. The possibility that hyperactive children have high lead levels because they are hyperactive, rather than vice versa, is not confounding; it is simply a case in which the direction of causality is turned around (effect-cause).

Lead-time bias refers to a distortion of the apparent efficacy of a screening program.

75–78.   The answers are: 75-A, 76-C, 77-B, 78-E. *(Mausner, ed 2. pp 47, 49, 55–56, 149–152, 312, 317.)* The *point prevalence* is the proportion of people in a population who have a disease at a given point in time. The numerator is the number of existing cases of a disease; the denominator is the total population at risk of the disease at that point in time.

In order to compare rates of disease or death in two or more groups that differ substantially in age, sex, or racial structure, adjustment or standardization of the rates is necessary to remove the effects of those differences. The *standardized mortality or morbidity ratio* (SMR) is the ratio of the observed number to the expected number of deaths or cases of the disease. For example, age-specific rates of angina pectoris in nonsmokers can be applied to the age distribution of smokers to obtain the expected number of cases of angina pectoris in the smokers. The SMR of smokers for angina pectoris is the observed number of cases divided by the expected number so calculated.

The *incidence rate* is the number of new cases of a disease that occur in a period of time divided by the population at risk during that time.

The *relative risk* is the incidence of disease in subjects with a risk factor divided by the incidence in those in whom the factor is absent. (The denominator is *not* the incidence in the general population because then subjects *with* the risk factor would be included. If the risk factor is uncommon and the relative risk is close to 1.0, the error involved in using the general population for the denominator is small. However, other risk factors, e.g., a relative with CHD, are quite prevalent.) The term *relative risk* can be confusing when the risk factor has to do with being a *relative* of a patient; in this instance *risk ratio* is a preferable synonym.

79–83.   The answers are: 79-C, 80-E, 81-D, 82-B, 83-A. *(Wilson, ed 12. p 7.)* Although these terms are usually applied to epidemiologic studies, they are also applicable to examples from everyday life. Lead-time bias commonly refers to the apparent increase in life expectancy seen in patients who have their disease diagnosed with a screening test. The problem is that the screening test does not actually result in the patients' living any longer than they would have otherwise; the fact is simply that these patients are detected with the disease earlier in the disease's course. The same would be true of a study that found that anatomy students lived at the same address for a longer period of time than fourth-year medical students, most of whom move to start internships. The study would not be wrong, but any conclusions that suggested that anatomy students are more stable than fourth-year clerks would be meaningless.

Surveillance bias refers to overdetection of the disease of interest because one of the groups goes to the doctor (or has a diagnostic test) more often than does another group. For example, women who take postmenopausal estrogens presumably go to the doctor (and probably have mammograms) more frequently than women who do not; thus, women who take estrogens may be more likely to have breast cancers detected because of the increased surveillance. Similarly, you are more likely to find something that is lost in June (when you may be moving) than in March, when you are presumably in the middle of the term.

Recall bias classically refers to a situation in which persons with a disease are more likely to remember an exposure (say, to a toxic chemical) than persons who are healthy. This is part of a human tendency to look for explanations for bad outcomes—like failing an examination.

A type 1 error occurs when a result is found to be statistically significant by chance in a sample even though there is no effect in the population. In the case of answering the question correctly, the chance of a type 1 error is 20 percent because even if you did not know anything about this question, you would have a 1 in 5 chance of getting it correct. This could also be an example of misclassification bias. Misclassification bias usually occurs when someone without a disease is mistakenly classified as having the disease (for example, someone who dies suddenly of a pulmonary embolism may be misclassified as having died of a myocardial infarction). It can also refer to misclassification of the exposure status of a person; for example, a nonsmoker might be classified as a smoker because he or she checked the wrong box on a form. Medical school faculty commonly misclassify students; your best hope is to try to ensure that the misclassification is in your favor.

Power is the chance of finding an effect in your sample if it truly exists in the population. One problem with finding out that your friends have been out at the movies is that they may not tell you the truth (recall bias), or you may ask the wrong ones, such as those sitting next to you in the library (surveillance bias). So you can give yourself credit if you made one of those choices as well, assuming you understood what you were doing!

84–87.   The answers are: 84-B, 85 E, 86-A, 87-C. *(Mausner, ed 2. pp 54–55, 264, 280–281.)* The *case-fatality rate* is a measure of the severity of the disease. It is a ratio of the number of deaths caused by a disease to the total number of cases of that disease and is usually expressed as a percentage. The *crude mortality* equals the total number of deaths from all causes during a year divided by the average population at risk during that year. It is usually expressed as the number of deaths per 1,000 people. The *secondary attack rate* is a measure of the contagiousness of an infectious disease. The numerator is the number of cases of disease occurring in contacts of the index case; the denominator is the number of contacts exposed to the index case during a specified period. Rates of disease are called *morbidity rates*.

88-91. The answers are: 88-A, 89-B, 90-B, 91-A. *(Ehrlich, Pediatrics 70:665, 1982. Siegel, pp 315-344.)* One of the most commonly made statistical errors is use of tests that assume that each of the observations is independent when data sets violate that assumption. Be very suspicious that this assumption might be violated any time the denominators are greater than the number of study subjects. For example, in question 88, even though group sizes were 24 and 9, denominators for the proportions compared were 231 and 55. If observations are independent, it means that each observation gives the same amount of information. For dichotomous (yes/no) variables, as in this example, it means that the probability of a "yes" is the same for each observation. Returning to the example of urine cultures, since the overall proportion of positive cultures was 34/55 in the diversion group, it means that the best estimate of the probability that each culture will be positive should be 34/55. But what if one particular patient had received 20 of those cultures, and 19 had been positive? The best estimate of the probability that another culture from that person would be positive is 19/20, not 34/55. Thus, if one wishes to estimate the probability of a positive culture in an individual, not all the observations in the sample give the same amount of information: previous cultures on the same person would be more informative than cultures on others.

The situation is similar (though a bit more subtle) in question 91. Here the denominators are (appropriately) children, but once again, not all observations are independent. The trouble here is that all the subjects are in four classrooms, and if one child in the class develops chickenpox, other children in that class are much more likely to do so. For example, if by chance the one new contact with chickenpox happened to be in one of the control group classes, many people in that class would be infected. As was the case with urine cultures, if one wanted to estimate the probability that a specific child would get chickenpox, not all observations would be equally informative; observations on other members of the same class would be much more relevant.

Another very commonly made error is use of statistics that assume that the data are normally distributed when that assumption is false. This is the error in questions 89 and 90. The normal distribution is bell-shaped, symmetric, and continuous. Data with a limited number of categories (such as parity) violate the assumption of normality, particularly if the mode is not somewhere near the middle category. The other main way in which the normality assumption is violated is by very skewed distributions, i.e., asymmetric distributions that have some very extreme values on one side. Length of hospital stay is a good example: A single patient with a very complicated hospital course may tremendously affect the mean length of stay and its standard deviation in whichever group that patient is in. (Note that to some extent, these two effects cancel each other out because they tend to affect the p value in opposite directions. The statistical way of saying this is that the t test is fairly *robust* to violations of the assumption of normality.) A helpful rule is this: There should be equal numbers of values at the mean plus and minus two standard deviations. In questions 89 and 90, values of < 1.0 or 1.5 standard deviations below the mean were not possible: a negative length of stay or a negative number of children would result. (In each case the mean is less than 2.0 standard deviations from a lower limit for the variable.) Whenever the assumption of normality is not reasonable, and the sample size is not large, the data should be analyzed using a nonparametric technique, such as a rank sum test. In the example regarding length of hospital stay, it is quite possible that use of a nonparametric technique would lead to a lower p value, if, for example, there were a few patients with very long lengths of stay, as might be expected in a study of premature infants. Note that the assumption of a normally distributed variable is most important when the sample size is small. With large sample sizes (N > 100), the t test can be used even with very skewed variables because the central limit theorem applies.

92–95. The answers are: 92-D, 93-A, 94-B, 95-D. *(Colton, pp 6–7, 243–244.)* For proper comparison of the frequency of a disease in two groups, the rate of disease, not the number of cases, must be compared. The number of cases may reflect the age structure of the population served by the hospital. Age-specific attack rates that incorporate the number of cases in each age group, divided by the number of persons in each group, should be calculated.

In order to determine that an association between two conditions such as diabetes and obesity exists, an investigator must show that obesity is significantly more common in persons who have diabetes than in persons who do not have diabetes. The controls are necessary in order to test the significance of the association and must resemble the cases as closely as possible in all ways except for the absence of the disease under study.

Whenever considerable numbers of a cohort are lost to follow-up, doubts about the validity of the conclusions arise. Because death may be a major reason for loss to follow-up, the most conservative approach is to assume that everyone lost to follow-up has died. Unless, in this example, the death rate in the anxiety neurosis cohort was *still* no greater than that in the general population (after adding another 50 deaths for the 20 percent of the 250 patients lost to follow-up), the conclusions are suspect.

The conclusion in question 95 is invalid because of the lack of denominators to calculate the rate of bacterial endocarditis in different age groups. In addition, the autopsy series merely gives an estimate of the proportion of deaths in different age groups, not the frequency of occurrence of endocarditis with age. The autopsy series may also be invalid as a source of data from which to draw conclusions because of factors that determined whether an autopsy was performed.

96–99. The answers are: 96-B, 97-A, 98-E, 99-B. *(Hulley, pp 99–108. Mausner, ed 2. pp 329–332.)* Matching is a way of selecting subjects that are comparable with respect to specific variables. For example, in a case-control study, a control could be selected that is the same age and sex as the case. It is thus a *sampling* strategy to achieve comparability among groups.

Stratification is an analysis strategy with the same purpose. Thus, after the study has been completed, the subjects can be stratified, i.e., divided into separate, relatively homogeneous strata, and the comparison between groups can occur within each stratum. For example, survival could be compared separately in different age strata, as in question 96. This might be important if the subjects with high renin levels were also older than the subjects with low levels, since a difference in survival between the two groups might be due to age, rather than to differing renin levels.

Age adjustment takes stratification by age one step further. After mortality (or another parameter) is calculated for specific age strata, it is combined in a weighted average to yield a single number. The weights used are the sizes of the different age strata in a standard population. Age adjustment is used most often for comparing mortality in populations with differing age structures.

Multivariate statistical analysis, like stratification, is an analysis technique for achieving comparability among groups. It involves *modeling* the associations between variables in order to allow their different effects to be isolated from each other. (For example, in multiple regression, the relationships between variables are modeled as a straight line.)

Survival analysis is a technique by which persons followed for variable lengths of time are counted according to the length of time they were followed. For example, in the cohort study of renin levels mentioned above, instead of simply comparing the proportions surviving 5 years, the cumulative probability of survival could be plotted for the two groups, and the two curves compared.

100-103.   The answers are: 100-A, 101-D, 102-E, 103-C. *(Hulley, pp 204-205.)*
If the probability of an event is p, the *odds* of the event are $p/(1-p)$. The *odds ratio* is the ratio of the odds of exposure to the risk factor given disease (a/c) to the odds of exposure to the risk factor given no disease (b/d). To illustrate that the odds of exposure given disease are a/c, the probability of exposure given disease is $p = a/(a+c)$. So $(1-p) = c/(a+c)$, and the odds are $[a/(a+c)]/[c/(a+c)]$, and the $(a+c)$'s cancel out to give a/c. The odds ratio, therefore, is $(a/c)/(b/d)$, which equals ad/bc.

Odds ratios are mainly used in case-control studies, from which relative risk cannot be calculated directly. When the disease is rare, the odds ratio closely approximates the relative risk. However, the study in the example is a cohort study, so relative risk can be calculated directly from the table. It is equal to the risk (incidence) of suicide in those who served in Vietnam divided by the risk in those who served elsewhere, or $[a/(a+b)]/[c/(c+d)]$.

Excess risk is defined as the *difference* between the risk in those with the risk factor and those in whom it is absent. Whereas the relative risk and odds ratio are unitless (since any measurement of time in the denominators cancels out), the excess risk must have an explicit or implied time period on the denominator. In this example, a/(a + b) − c/(c + d) represents the excess risk of suicide in Vietnam veterans over a 5-year period; it is five times as big as the excess risk for a 1-year period. Thus, if the yearly risk of suicide was 0.2 percent in Vietnam veterans and 0.1 percent in other veterans, the relative risk would be 2.0, and the excess risk (risk difference) 0.1 percent per year, or 0.5 percent over the 5-year period.

The overall incidence of suicide (per 5 years) in the study is simply the number of suicides (a + c) divided by the population at risk (a + b + c + d). (Note that a more precise way to measure the incidence, relative risk, and so on would be to use person-years at risk on the denominators, but this leads to greater computational and conceptual complexity.)

104–107.   The answers are: 104-C, 105-E, 106-A, 107-D. *(Hulley, pp 24–25.)* *Simple random sampling* is a process in which individuals are sampled independently, and each individual of the population has an equal probability of being selected.

In *cluster sampling*, groups of people (e.g., families, school classes) are selected at random, and then everyone in those groups is sampled. A common analytic mistake is to pretend that subjects obtained in a cluster sample were obtained in a simple random sample. This can lead to incorrect results because the subjects are not sampled independently.

Systematic sampling is a process that first requires the arrangement of the group to be sampled in some kind of order. Then individuals are selected systematically throughout the series on the basis of a predetermined sampling fraction or constant determinant, for example, every fifth, tenth, or hundredth person in the ordered group. Although systematic sampling may seem almost the same as simple random sampling, it is much less desirable. For example, sampling every other subject from a list in which husbands' and wives' names appear next to each other (e.g., an alphabetical list) will bias the sample—if husbands were always first, the sample might include no wives and would rarely include both persons in a married couple.

In *stratified sampling*, a population is divided into subgroups based on defined characteristics such as age, sex, or severity of illness, or any combination of these; then random samples are selected from each subgroup.

In *paired sampling*, or *matching*, selection of one or more controls for each case is based on age, sex, time, time sequence, geographic location, or some other defined relationship to the case. For example, selection could be based on the next patient admitted after each case, the sibling nearest in age to each case, or the person who lives closest geographically to each case.

108–112.   The answers are: 108-D, 109-E, 110-B, 111-E, 112-E. *(Wilson, ed 12. p 7.)* The easiest (and best) way to answer problems like this is to write out the appropriate two-by-two table. Since we were not told how many women were tested, we can just make up a number—say, 200. We are told that half have a positive test:

	Infection	No Infection	
Test Positive	?	?	100
Test Negative	?	?	100
			200

The next task is to fill in the remaining boxes. We are told that 45 percent of those with a positive test are infected with chlamydia:

	Infection	No Infection	
Test Positive	45	55	100
Test Negative	?	?	100
			200

and that 95 percent of those with a negative test are free of the disease:

	Infection	No Infection	
Test Positive	45	55	100
Test Negative	5	95	100
			200

This now allows us to say that for 200 women in the community, the following two-by-two table would be correct:

	Infection	No Infection	
Test Positive	45	55	100
Test Negative	5	95	100
	50	150	200

We can now determine the test's operating characteristics (sensitivity and specificity) and the other parameters. Sensitivity is simply the proportion of women with chlamydia who will have a positive test (remember: *PID* = *P*ositivity *i*n *D*isease), or $45/50 = 90$ percent. Specificity is the proportion of women without chlamydia who will have a negative test (remember: *NIH* = *N*egativity *i*n *H*ealth), or $95/150 = 63$ percent. The prevalence of the disease is simply the proportion of women with chlamydia, or 50 out of $200 = 25$ percent. The predictive value of a positive test is the proportion of women with a positive test who have chlamydia; we were already told that this was 45 percent. Likewise, the predictive value of a negative test is the proportion of women with a negative test who do not have chlamydia; we were already told that this was 95 percent.

113–116.   The answers are: 113-B, 114-D, 115-A, 116-E. *(Colton, pp 28-31.)* Mean, median, and mode are all measures of central tendency, while variance, standard deviation, and range are measures of dispersion. In figure B, both distributions appear normally shaped, and they center on the same point, but curve 2 has greater variance because it is more spread out. Figure D, in contrast, shows two distributions with the same variance, but different means. In figure A, both the centers and the shapes of the curves differ. Curve 1 is skewed to the right, which means it has more of a tail on the right side.

Remember that the value that occurs most commonly (i.e., the highest point on the curve) is the mode, so choice E represents "pi a la mode"—a very tasty dessert.

117–120.   The answers are: 117-C, 118-A, 119-B, 120-D. *(Browner, JAMA 257:2459-2463, 1987. Michael, pp 31-38, 91-95, 105-112.)* A type 2 error occurs when a study fails to reject the null hypothesis (of no effect), when it is in fact false. Any time a study fails to achieve statistical significance, a crucial question to ask is whether the study had enough subjects. Although 500 subjects per group followed for 5 years seems like a large number, only a tiny minority (perhaps 10 per group) would be expected to have a myocardial infarction. Thus the sample size in this instance may have been inadequate to detect a meaningful difference between the groups.

The ecologic fallacy occurs when associations among groups of subjects are mistakenly assumed to hold for individuals. Thus, although among communities high rates of condom use may be associated with higher fertility rates (perhaps because condom use acts as a marker for sexual activity in general), among those who use the condoms, the fertility rate could in fact be zero.

A type 1 error occurs when, just by chance, a statistically significant difference between groups is found. Studies attempting to correlate multiple risk factors with multiple diseases (particularly when there is no good biologic reason to suspect an association) are especially prone to type 1 errors. Looking for associations separately in different subgroups compounds the problem.

Selection bias occurs when the subjects selected for the study are somehow not representative of the population from which they come. One trouble with selecting spouses for controls is that one's spouse is much more likely to share one's smoking habits than a person from the general population. Thus, since patients with lung cancer will be mostly smokers, smokers will be overrepresented among the controls, and smoking will look like a weaker risk factor than it really is.

121–125.   The answers are: 121-A, 122-C, 123-E, 124-B, 125-D. *(Last, ed 2. p 80.)* The scale of measurement is an important determinant of the amount of information in a variable and the type of statistical analysis that can be used. Dichotomous variables (like sex) have only two possible values. Some variables may be artificially dichotomized, with subsequent loss of information. For example, a patient either survives 5 years or not; thus survival to 5 years is an example of a dichotomous variable. The variable could be made more informative, however, if the actual number of months of survival was specified.

Nominal variables have more than two possible values, but no intrinsic ordering. Race is the classic example; medical specialties also have no intrinsic ordering. Nominal and ordinal are often confused. Just remember *no*minal for *no* ordering.

Ordinal variables are intrinsically ordered, but not in a quantitative way that allows one to say that there is a natural numerical distance between possible values. Thus one value cannot really be subtracted from another. Examples are qualitative judgments like "worse, same, better" or "never, sometimes, always." Remember, *ordi*nal means *order*ed.

Interval scales are ordered, but with real numerical units; they can be subtracted from each other. An example is dates of birth: they are intrinsically ordered and subtracting them gives meaningful numbers, but there is no intrinsic zero to the scale, so that dividing them does not make a lot of sense—one date of birth cannot be twice as big as another.

Ratio scales are measurements in relation to a clear zero point. Thus, measurements on ratio scales can be meaningfully divided by each other. For example, one baby may weigh twice as much as another, or have twice as high a platelet count. Absolute temperature is measured on a ratio scale, whereas temperature in Fahrenheit or Celsius is measured on an interval scale.

126–130.   The answers are: 126–A, 127–A, 128–A, 129–E, 130–D. *(Sackett, pp 59–100.)* Answering the first three of these questions is easiest if the results of Dr. Blues' research are displayed in a two-by-two table:

	Depressed	Not Depressed
Positive Blues test	80	80
Negative Blues test	20	320
Total	100	400

The sensitivity of a test is defined as the proportion of persons with a disease who have a positive test (positivity in disease = PID): in this case, 80 out of 100, or 80 percent. This is the same as the likelihood that a person with depression will have a positive Blues test. The specificity of a test is defined as the proportion of persons without a disease who have a negative test (negativity in health = NIH): in this case, 320 out of 400, or 80 percent.

The likelihood that someone with a positive test has the disease—known as the positive predictive value (PV+) of a test—depends upon how prevalent the disease is. By definition,

PV+ = true positives ÷ total positives
     = true positives ÷ (true positives + false positives)
     = (sensitivity × prevalence) ÷ [(sensitivity × prevalence)
       + (1 − specificity) × (1 − prevalence)]
     = (0.8 × 0.01) ÷ [(0.8 × 0.01) + (0.2 × 0.99)] = 3.9%

The Blues test would not be very useful in diagnosing depression if applied to the general population. It might be useful in ruling out depression if negative, however. The likelihood that someone with a negative test has the disease equals 100 percent minus the likelihood that someone with a negative test does *not* have the disease. This latter quantity is known as the negative predictive value (PV−) and is defined as

PV− = true negatives ÷ total negatives
     = true negatives ÷ (true negatives + false negatives)
     = [specificity × (1 − prevalence)] ÷ [specificity × (1 − prevalence)
       + (1 − sensitivity × prevalence)]
     = (0.8 × 0.99) ÷ [(0.8 × 0.99) + (0.2 × 0.01)] = 99.7%

Since the likelihood that someone with a negative test is *not* depressed is 99.7 percent, the likelihood that someone with a negative test is depressed is (1 − 99.7 percent) or 0.3 percent. (A shortcut: Since we know that the overall prevalence of depression is only 1 percent, someone with a *negative* Blues test must be even less likely to be depressed than that!)

Epidemiology of
Health and Disease

c ε c β

DIRECTIONS: Each question below contains five suggested responses. Select the **one best** response to each question.

131. Which of the following statements about aortic dissection is true?

(A) Almost all patients with aortic dissection have elevated serum cholesterol levels (> 240 mg/dL)
(B) Aortic dissection is the major cause of mortality in patients with Marfan's syndrome
(C) There is an increased incidence of aortic dissection in patients with Gaucher's disease
(D) There is approximately a 10 percent operative mortality from emergency surgery for dissection of the ascending aorta
(E) Acute aortic dissection is usually asymptomatic

132. The incidence of nosocomial infections among patients admitted to general hospitals in the United States is about

(A) 1 percent
(B) 3 percent
(C) 6 percent
(D) 12 percent
(E) 18 percent

133. In country A there are 35 new cases of breast cancer per 100,000 adult women per year; in country B the number is 90 per 100,000. Which of the following is the most likely explanation?

(A) Women in country A have a much higher rate of nursing their infants
(B) Women in country A are less likely to smoke cigarettes
(C) Women in country A receive more frequent preventive care, such as mammography
(D) Treatment is much more successful in country A
(E) Women in country A are younger

134. Studies in the epidemiology of appendicitis have shown that

(A) it affects girls nearly three times as frequently as boys
(B) its incidence is highest in the sixth and seventh decades of life
(C) its incidence is decreasing in the Western world
(D) its mortality is increasing in the Western world
(E) it affects about 1 in 1,000 pregnancies

135. Correct statements about infant mortality include which of the following?

(A) The numerator is the number of deaths of infants in the first month of life
(B) The rate is expressed per 1,000 births
(C) In the U.S., the single most important cause of infant mortality is sudden infant death syndrome (SIDS)
(D) In the U.S., infant mortality is about twice as high in blacks as in whites
(E) None of the above

136. True statements about complications of appendicitis include all the following EXCEPT

(A) there is at least a 70 percent incidence of appendiceal perforation among patients with appendicitis who are under 2 years of age
(B) there is a 30 percent incidence of appendiceal perforation among patients with appendicitis who are over 70 years of age
(C) the incidence of perforation is higher in patients with leukocytosis (> 20,000 cells per microliter)
(D) surgical mortality is about 0.1 percent in the absence of perforation
(E) surgical mortality is about twice as high in the presence of perforation

137. Chickenpox is associated with

(A) a high case fatality rate
(B) congenital malformations in 10 percent of offspring of infected mothers
(C) a high reinfection rate
(D) a long prodromal period
(E) Reye syndrome

138. Giardiasis occurs on a worldwide basis and is associated with all the following EXCEPT

(A) waterborne transmission
(B) asymptomatic carriage
(C) bloating, abdominal cramps, and diarrhea
(D) invasion of colonic mucosa
(E) transmission from person to person

139. The newborn with cytomegalovirus (CMV) infection at birth most commonly presents with

(A) hepatosplenomegaly
(B) hepatitis
(C) thrombocytopenia
(D) cerebral calcifications
(E) no symptoms

140. Factors that are more characteristic of childhood-onset asthma than adult-onset asthma include

(A) a 2:1 ratio of females to males
(B) an association with a history of eczema
(C) normal levels of IgE in the serum
(D) lack of response to provocation with inhaled antigens
(E) lack of seasonal variation in severity of symptoms

141. Which of the following bacteria is the most common cause of bacterial meningitis in children 3 months to 6 years of age in the United States?

(A) *Streptococcus pneumoniae*
(B) *Neisseria meningitidis*
(C) *Haemophilus influenzae* type b
(D) *Escherichia coli* K1
(E) Group B *Streptococcus hemolyticus*

142. The bacteria that are involved in nosocomial (hospital-associated) infections are transmitted most often by

(A) airborne matter
(B) fomites
(C) exposure to a common source
(D) indwelling catheters
(E) direct contact via hands

143. All the following are clearly associated with acute episodes of asthma EXCEPT

(A) emotional stress
(B) elevated ozone concentrations
(C) glaucoma therapy
(D) alcohol
(E) upper respiratory infections

144. Between 50 and 60 percent of fatal motor vehicle accidents in the United States are caused by drunk drivers, according to the Insurance Institute for Highway Safety. The most effective means to date of reducing drunk driving is

(A) heavy fine
(B) mandatory jail sentence
(C) rehabilitation program
(D) restitution
(E) suspension of license

145. Which is the most common site of nosocomial infections?

(A) Surgical wound
(B) Respiratory tract
(C) Skin
(D) Urinary tract
(E) Gastrointestinal tract

146. Compared with Western European countries (excluding Northern Ireland), the homicide rate in the U.S. is

(A) about 25 percent lower
(B) about the same
(C) about 50 percent higher
(D) two to three times as high
(E) about ten times as high

147. A major complication of transfusion of blood and blood products has been the development of posttransfusion hepatitis. Research indicates that

(A) most cases of posttransfusion hepatitis are due to infection with hepatitis B virus
(B) the risk of posttransfusion hepatitis is highest following transfusions of albumin or immune globulin
(C) about 5 to 10 percent of patients who received blood or blood products developed posttransfusion hepatitis
(D) no screening test is available to detect blood that may transmit hepatitis C virus
(E) almost all cases of posttransfusion hepatitis are asymptomatic

148. Correct statements about obesity include all the following EXCEPT

(A) a woman whose body fat is equal to 24 percent of her total body weight should be considered obese

(B) obesity is the major risk factor for non-insulin-dependent diabetes mellitus

(C) sedentariness is the most important cause of widespread obesity in Western populations

(D) obesity is a risk factor for coronary heart disease only among the extremely obese

(E) genetic factors contribute to obesity

149. True statements about the epidemiology of cancer in the U.S., excluding nonmelanoma skin cancers and cancer in situ, include all the following EXCEPT

(A) about 1 million cases of cancer develop each year

(B) cancer is responsible for about 25 percent of deaths

(C) one in three Americans will develop cancer in his or her lifetime

(D) the 5-year survival with cancer is about 50 percent

(E) mortality from lung cancer has declined steadily since 1975

150. The parameter that can be used to obtain the best estimate of the prevalence of dental caries is

(A) the calculus index

(B) the malocclusion index

(C) the decayed, missing, or filled rate

(D) the oral hygiene index

(E) none of the above

151. Correct statements concerning upper respiratory infections include which of the following?

(A) Summertime outbreaks of illness characterized by fever, pharyngitis, and conjunctivitis have most frequently been associated with paramyxovirus infection

(B) Treatment with penicillin hastens recovery in children with streptococcal pharyngitis

(C) Patients with viral upper respiratory infections are generally most infectious the day before their symptoms begin

(D) The most common identifiable cause of pharyngitis is adenovirus

(E) None of the above

152. Studies of coronary artery bypass grafting have shown that all the following are true EXCEPT

(A) operative mortality is higher in women than in men

(B) operative mortality is higher in persons with diabetes

(C) operative mortality is approximately 1 percent in persons with normal left ventricular function

(D) when adjusted for severity of disease, there is little variation in operative mortality for surgery performed by different board-certified surgeons

(E) surgery reduces or eliminates angina in about 85 percent of patients

153. Which statement about obesity is correct?

(A) Osteoarthritis is less common among obese persons because of decreased activity
(B) In a normal person, 300 calories of excess carbohydrate will lead to the same weight gain as 300 calories of excess fat
(C) Obese persons are significantly less active than nonobese persons
(D) The apparent association between obesity and hypertension is probably due to the use of inappropriately small blood pressure cuffs in the obese subjects
(E) None of the above

154. Correct statements concerning breast-feeding include which of the following?

(A) The incidence of infections is greater in breast-fed than in bottle-fed infants
(B) Breast milk is frequently insufficient in quantity
(C) Iron deficiency anemia is less frequent in infants fed cow's milk than in breast-fed infants
(D) Significant quantities of immunoglobulins are provided by breast milk
(E) None of the above

155. Overconsumption of refined sugar has been shown to cause

(A) obesity
(B) arteriosclerosis
(C) diabetes
(D) parotitis
(E) none of the above

156. All the following statements about coronary heart disease in the U.S. are true EXCEPT

(A) about 5 million Americans have coronary heart disease
(B) coronary heart disease is the leading cause of death in men 35 to 44 years of age
(C) among the elderly, angina is a more frequent presentation in women than in men
(D) the incidence of coronary heart disease increases fivefold from 40 to 60 years of age in both men and women
(E) coronary heart disease is the second most common cause of death in women of all ages

157. Which of the following statements about colon cancer in the U.S. is true?

(A) It is two times more common in smokers
(B) It is the second leading cause of cancer death in males
(C) It is a rare cause of cancer death in women
(D) There is an increased incidence of the disease in alcoholics
(E) The death rate from the disease has been decreasing steadily for the past 20 years

158. Among patients with intermittent claudication, all the following statements are true EXCEPT

(A) about 50 percent eventually require amputation if they do not undergo vascular reconstruction
(B) the leading cause of death is coronary heart disease
(C) about 50 percent have significant coronary artery disease at the time of presentation
(D) prognosis is worse in patients with diabetes
(E) the 10-year survival after presentation is about 50 percent

159. Which of the following epidemiologic statements about gastric cancer is true?

(A) The incidence of gastric cancer is higher in Japan than in the U.S.
(B) Annual mortality for gastric cancer has been increasing over the last 40 years in the U.S.
(C) The incidence of gastric cancer is higher in smokers
(D) The incidence in women is twice that in men
(E) The incidence is higher in persons with a history of benign gastric ulcer

160. Premature loss of life can be defined as years of life lost due to a disease before the age of 65 years. The leading cause of premature loss of life in the U.S. is

(A) coronary heart disease
(B) cancer
(C) stroke
(D) congenital heart disease
(E) none of the above

161. All the following statements about blindness are true EXCEPT

(A) cataracts cause between one-third and one-half of the cases of blindness in the third world
(B) glaucoma is the most important cause of blindness among blacks in the U.S.
(C) persons with severe myopia are at an increased risk of retinal detachment
(D) proliferative retinopathy is the most common cause of blindness among persons with type I (juvenile-onset, insulin-dependent) diabetes
(E) trachoma is the most common cause of retinal detachment worldwide

162. Compared with the general population, all the following patients are at an increased risk of cobalamin (B_{12}) deficiency EXCEPT

(A) a 40-year-old man with a history of ingestion of lye at age 20
(B) a 20-year-old woman with a history of Graves' disease
(C) a 60-year-old man with a brother with pernicious anemia
(D) a 70-year-old woman with a nematodal infection
(E) a 30-year-old man with Crohn's disease

163. Which of the following statements about microcytic anemia in the U.S. is true?

(A) It usually has a genetic cause in black children
(B) It is rarely caused by a dietary deficiency in men
(C) It is rarely caused by a dietary deficiency in women
(D) It is more common in formula-fed than breast-fed infants
(E) It is not associated with pica

164. All the following are independently associated with poor prognosis in colon cancer EXCEPT

(A) size of the tumor
(B) preoperative carcinoembryonic antigen (CEA) titer
(C) number of involved lymph nodes
(D) poorly differentiated histology
(E) tumor in pericolonic fat

165. The ratio of the prevalence of type I (insulin-dependent) diabetes mellitus to type II (non-insulin-dependent) diabetes mellitus in the U.S. is about

(A) 1:1
(B) 1:4
(C) 1:9
(D) 4:1
(E) 9:1

166. A characteristic demographic feature of rheumatoid arthritis is an incidence ratio of 1:3 that applies to

(A) male:female
(B) blacks:whites
(C) rural:urban inhabitants
(D) high:low socioeconomic status
(E) Western:Eastern cultures

167. Possible risk factors for the development of colon cancer include all the following EXCEPT

(A) diets high in animal fat
(B) irritable bowel syndrome
(C) inflammatory bowel disease
(D) familial polyposis
(E) ureterosigmoidostomy

168. Which of the following statements about valvular heart disease is true?

(A) Coronary artery disease is the most common cause of aortic stenosis in the U.S.
(B) The incidence of rheumatic heart disease in the U.S. has been rising for the past 10 years
(C) Most persons with a history of rheumatic fever are immune to recurrences during group A streptococcal epidemics
(D) Most cases of mitral valve prolapse are asymptomatic
(E) None of the above

169. Cystic fibrosis is a genetic disorder of eccrine and exocrine gland function. All the following statements about cystic fibrosis are true EXCEPT

(A) it is the most common genetic disease in whites in the U.S.
(B) it is inherited as an autosomal recessive trait
(C) about 1 in 20 whites are heterozygous for the gene
(D) the diagnosis can be confirmed by demonstrating an absence of chloride in the sweat
(E) about 50 percent of patients survive beyond age 15

170. Asthma is characterized by which of the following?

(A) Age of onset before age 40 in about 95 percent of cases
(B) Persistently abnormal forced expiratory volume in 1 s (FEV_1)
(C) Greater frequency in girls than boys
(D) Frequent family history of atopy
(E) None of the above

171. The epidemiology of cystic fibrosis indicates that

(A) about 1 in 200 white Americans carries the gene responsible for the disease
(B) there is an increased gene frequency among the Amish
(C) antenatal diagnosis is not possible
(D) median survival after birth is about 8 years
(E) about 40 percent of men with cystic fibrosis are infertile

172. Which of the following statements about emphysema is true?

(A) There is a definitive clinical diagnosis of the disease
(B) Cigarette smokers are twice as likely to develop the disease as nonsmokers
(C) Flow rates on pulmonary function tests resemble those seen in chronic bronchitis
(D) It is equally prevalent in light and heavy smokers
(E) It is associated with the chronic inhalation of coal dust

173. Studies of estimated mortality related to birth control in premenopausal women have shown that

(A) at all ages, mortality is greater among women using no contraception than among women using oral contraceptives
(B) the mortality among women ages 40 to 44 associated with the use of abortion is less than one-twentieth that associated with birth
(C) death rates associated with the use of intrauterine devices (IUDs) are about ten times higher in older than in younger women
(D) smokers who use birth control pills are at about a 15 percent higher mortality risk
(E) the highest birth-related death rates are seen among teen-agers

174. Studies of musculoskeletal disorders in the U.S. have found that all the following statements are true EXCEPT

(A) they are a more common cause of limitation of activity than is cardiovascular disease
(B) back or spine impairments are the most common type
(C) from 60 to 80 percent of the population experiences back pain at some time during their lives
(D) persons who engage in heavy manual work have a greater risk of suffering low back pain than persons who work at sedentary jobs
(E) lower back x-rays and medical examinations are useful ways to screen for workers at high risk of sustaining on-the-job back injuries

175. Which of the following statements about bronchiectasis is true?

(A) It is uncommon in childhood
(B) It is manifested by cough
(C) It is rarely accompanied by fever
(D) It is usually a primary disorder
(E) It is usually a self-limited problem

176. Studies of the epidemiology of cutaneous drug reactions have shown which of the following?

(A) The incidence of cutaneous drug reactions is highest in the elderly
(B) Urticaria is the most common skin manifestation
(C) Cutaneous drug reactions usually occur about 2 to 3 weeks following initial exposure
(D) The most common drugs involved are antihypertensive medications
(E) None of the above

177. International studies of cardiovascular disease have shown which of the following?

(A) Death rates due to coronary artery disease vary by less than 25 percent from country to country
(B) The death rate due to coronary artery disease is higher in the U.S. than in any European country
(C) The death rate due to coronary artery disease is similar in the U.S. and Japan
(D) The death rate due to coronary artery disease has been decreasing more rapidly in the U.S. than in any other country
(E) None of the above

178. Which of the following patients is most likely to have a stroke within a year?

(A) A 70-year-old male smoker with hypertension
(B) A 70-year-old female smoker with hypertension
(C) A 50-year-old woman with mitral valve prolapse
(D) A 50-year-old woman with a recent transient ischemic attack
(E) A 50-year-old man with an asymptomatic carotid bruit

179. Which of the following statements about elderly Americans is true?

(A) Most of the difference in life expectancy between men and women is due to unalterable genetic factors
(B) Although there are more elderly women than men, fewer elderly women live alone
(C) A woman is less likely to be institutionalized in a nursing home than is a man
(D) The number of persons older than 65 years of age is expected to increase by nearly 15 percent in the next 40 years
(E) None of the above

180. The incidence of cholelithiasis (gallstones) is increased in all the following EXCEPT

(A) persons with diabetes
(B) persons with chronic hemolytic anemia
(C) persons with hypercholesterolemia
(D) persons who are obese
(E) women

181. Which of the following statements about systemic lupus erythematosus (SLE) is true?

(A) It is more common in whites than blacks
(B) The incidence increases with age
(C) It is approximately ten times more common in women than men
(D) The diagnosis requires a positive antinuclear antibody (ANA) test
(E) It is the most common cause of arthritis in women less than 35 years of age

182. Compared with the general population, all the following patients are at an increased risk of folate deficiency EXCEPT

(A) a 20-year-old man with sickle cell anemia
(B) a 20-year-old woman who is a strict vegetarian
(C) a 60-year-old man on hemodialysis
(D) a 70-year-old woman who drinks a quart of vodka each day
(E) a 30-year-old man with tropical sprue

183. Compared with persons without kidney disease, patients on chronic dialysis for renal failure have an increased incidence of all the following EXCEPT

(A) infection with *Mycobacterium tuberculosis*
(B) infection with hepatitis B
(C) suicide
(D) coronary heart disease
(E) hypernephroma

184. The risk of developing cataracts is increased among all the following persons EXCEPT those

(A) who have type I (insulin-dependent) diabetes
(B) with a history of congenital rubella
(C) who have type II (non-insulin-dependent) diabetes
(D) with an occupational exposure to video display terminals
(E) with an occupational exposure to ultraviolet radiation

185. Which of the following is a risk factor for the development of hemophilia?

(A) HLA-B15
(B) Iron deficiency
(C) Hepatitis B surface antigen (HBsAg)
(D) Benzene exposure
(E) None of the above

186. Which of the following cancers has been associated with increasing age-adjusted mortality in the past 25 years?

(A) Lung cancer
(B) Uterine cancer
(C) Prostate cancer
(D) Scrotal cancer
(E) Stomach cancer

187. Primary hepatocellular carcinoma (hepatoma) is

(A) more common in persons with chronic liver disease
(B) associated with the consumption of raw meat
(C) responsible for 2 to 4 percent of all deaths from cancer in Africa
(D) associated with cigarette smoking
(E) more common in persons with gallstones

188. Seroepidemiologic studies of infection with herpes simplex virus (HSV) have shown that

(A) infection with HSV-2 is more common than infection with HSV-1
(B) the prevalence of antibodies to HSV-2 is more than five times higher than the reported history of infection
(C) HSV-2 is only infectious during the symptomatic phase
(D) it is possible to differentiate HSV-1 from HSV-2 antibodies
(E) genital HSV-2 infection is less likely to reactivate than genital HSV-1 infection

189. A familial aggregation pattern exists for cancer of all the following organs EXCEPT

(A) breast
(B) cervix
(C) stomach
(D) colon
(E) larynx

190. All the following statements about the relationship between marital status and cancer are true EXCEPT

(A) the risk of cancer of the cervix is higher in married women compared with single women
(B) the risk of cancer of the cervix is lower in women who marry late in life than in women who marry earlier
(C) the risk of breast cancer is higher in single than in married women
(D) the risk of ovarian cancer is not related to marital status
(E) the risk of cancer of the testes is higher in married than in single men

191. When describing the epidemiology of lung cancer in the U.S. in 1990, all the following statements are true EXCEPT

(A) lung cancer is the leading cause of cancer death in men and women
(B) the 5-year survival rate from lung cancer is less than 20 percent
(C) more than 50 percent of patients have metastatic disease at the time of initial presentation
(D) the incidence of lung cancer in men is increasing
(E) the incidence of lung cancer in women is increasing

192. Cigarette smoking increases the risk of acquiring cancers of all the following EXCEPT

(A) esophagus
(B) pancreas
(C) larynx and oral cavity
(D) bladder and kidney
(E) liver

193. Multiple sclerosis (MS) is a chronic demyelinating disease characterized by an increased incidence in all the following EXCEPT

(A) women
(B) persons with certain HLA types
(C) persons who live further from the equator
(D) blood relatives of persons with the disease
(E) blacks

194. All the following are associated with a poor prognosis in patients with pneumococcal pneumonia EXCEPT

(A) leukocytosis
(B) positive blood culture
(C) infection with type 3 pneumococcus
(D) patient's age less than 1 year
(E) meningitis

195. Worldwide decreases in incidence have been observed in which type of cancer?

(A) Leukemia
(B) Cancer of the cervix
(C) Cancer of the colon
(D) Cancer of the prostate
(E) Cancer of the breast

196. The incidence of skin cancer

(A) is unaffected by environmental factors
(B) increases with age
(C) is higher in alcoholics
(D) is higher in persons who live far from the equator
(E) is higher in women

197. The reasons for the poor 5-year survival rate for pancreatic cancer include all the following EXCEPT

(A) the difficulty of establishing a diagnosis early during pathogenesis
(B) the usual ineffectiveness of radiotherapy
(C) the usual ineffectiveness of chemotherapy
(D) the unsuitability of about 85 percent of patients for resection at the time of diagnosis
(E) underlying diseases such as diabetes mellitus

198. Disorders of the prostate gland are a major cause of morbidity and mortality among elderly men. All the following statements about these disorders are true EXCEPT

(A) by age 70, almost 30 percent of men have benign prostatic hypertrophy
(B) about 10 percent of men will eventually undergo surgery for benign prostatic hypertrophy
(C) prostate cancer is the third most common cause of cancer death among men in the U.S.
(D) prostate cancer is usually asymptomatic
(E) the incidence of prostate cancer is higher in blacks than in whites

199 All the following are associated with an increased risk of pulmonary thromboembolism EXCEPT

(A) hip fracture
(B) obesity
(C) surgery
(D) use of oral contraceptives
(E) hypertension

200. Although the etiology of adult rheumatoid arthritis is not known, studies of its epidemiology have shown that

(A) the incidence is 20 times higher in women than in men
(B) progressive joint destruction occurs in less than 20 percent of cases
(C) the vast majority of cases have their onset between the ages of 35 and 50
(D) there is no genetic predisposition to the disease
(E) there is an increased incidence of the disease in miners

201. True statements about osteo-arthritis (degenerative joint disease) include

(A) it is more than twice as common among women as men of the same age
(B) the pattern of joint involvement is essentially identical in all races among persons of the same age
(C) about 50 percent of persons over age 75 have some degenerative joint disease
(D) hereditary factors are important in Heberden's nodes
(E) none of the above

202. The probability that an asymp-tomatic person will suffer a stroke is increased with which of the following?

(A) A history of frequent headaches
(B) Alcoholism
(C) Electrocardiographic evidence of heart enlargement
(D) A type A personality
(E) None of the above

203. Factors associated with a poor prognosis in rheumatoid arthritis include all the following EXCEPT

(A) female sex
(B) high titers of rheumatoid factor
(C) subcutaneous nodules
(D) radiographic erosion on initial hand films
(E) symmetric arthritis

204. The use of oral contraceptives increases the risk of

(A) breast cancer
(B) vaginal cancer
(C) osteoporosis
(D) thromboembolism
(E) none of the above

205. Though much is still unknown about adult-onset diabetes mellitus, constitutional and environmental factors associated with an increased incidence of the disease include all the following EXCEPT

(A) obesity
(B) age
(C) family history of diabetes
(D) pregnancy
(E) occupation

206. Which of the following factors may contribute to development of chronic bronchitis?

(A) Use of nasal spray
(B) Altitude
(C) Occupation
(D) Alcohol abuse
(E) None of the above

207. Studies of the epidemiology of epilepsy have shown that

(A) brain tumor is the most common cause in children less than 12 years of age
(B) cerebrovascular disease is the most common cause in adults older than 50 years of age
(C) 20 to 25 percent of children will have one or more seizures with febrile illnesses at some time in their childhood
(D) 90 percent of patients with post-traumatic seizures require long-term anticonvulsant therapy
(E) seizures are more likely with rapidly growing malignancies, like glioblastomas

208. Complications of diabetes mellitus include all the following EXCEPT

(A) blindness
(B) pancreatic cancer
(C) limb loss
(D) myocardial infarction
(E) stroke

209. Epidemiologic investigations of testicular cancer have shown that

(A) the peak incidence occurs within 1 to 2 years of puberty
(B) there is an increased incidence in males with cryptorchidism
(C) there is an increased risk in males with a history of venereal disease
(D) there is an increased incidence in males with a family history of breast cancer
(E) there is no increased risk in males with a history of mumps orchitis

210. Exposure of nonsmokers to secondhand cigarette smoke may result in all the following EXCEPT

(A) increased incidence of osteoarthritis
(B) elevation of blood concentration of carbon monoxide
(C) increased incidence of lower respiratory tract infections during the first year of life
(D) eye irritation, headache, nasal congestion, cough
(E) exacerbation of chronic obstructive lung disease

211. Prognosis in Hodgkin's disease correlates with all the following EXCEPT

(A) the stage of disease at the time of diagnosis
(B) the presence of systemic symptoms
(C) the histologic type
(D) the sex of the patient
(E) HLA type

212. Among the following health care workers, the lowest prevalence of hepatitis B virus markers is found in

(A) dialysis staff
(B) blood bank technicians
(C) staff of custodial institutions for the mentally retarded
(D) surgical house staff
(E) medical house staff

213. The incidence of ulcerative colitis in the U.S. is approximately 6 per 100,000 per year; the prevalence is about 100 per 100,000. The incidence of Crohn's disease in the U.S. is approximately 2 per 100,000 per year; the prevalence is about 30 per 100,000. The incidences of both diseases are higher in whites than in blacks, with an odds ratio of 2.0. Duration of the disease is similar in whites and blacks. This implies that in the U.S.

(A) the incidence of Crohn's disease in whites is about 5 per 100,000 per year
(B) the prevalence of ulcerative colitis in blacks is about 90 per 100,000
(C) the average duration of Crohn's disease is similar to that of ulcerative colitis
(D) the odds ratio is not a valid measure of the relative risk for these diseases
(E) there are approximately 15,000 persons in the U.S. with ulcerative colitis

214. Exposure to benzene has been associated with all the following hematologic diseases EXCEPT

(A) aplastic anemia
(B) non-Hodgkin lymphoma
(C) acute nonlymphocytic leukemia
(D) acute lymphocytic leukemia
(E) chronic myelogenous leukemia

215. The development of neuropathic symptoms is associated with chronic exposure to all the following substances EXCEPT

(A) mercury
(B) lead
(C) arsenic
(D) sulfur dioxide
(E) nitrous oxide

216. Which one of the following diseases is found almost exclusively among persons who have worked with or have been exposed to asbestos?

(A) Bronchogenic carcinoma
(B) Byssinosis
(C) Pleural mesothelioma
(D) Laryngeal carcinoma
(E) Alveolar cell carcinoma

217. All the following chemicals have been associated with kidney disease EXCEPT

(A) β-naphthylamine
(B) cadmium
(C) ethylene glycol
(D) halogenated hydrocarbons
(E) lead

218. Which one of the following is the major cause of skin cancer due to occupational exposure?

(A) Anthracene
(B) Coal tar
(C) Creosote oil
(D) Radium and roentgen rays
(E) Ultraviolet light

219. Which of the following substances is causally associated with pneumoconiosis?

(A) Sulfur oxides
(B) Nitrogen oxides
(C) Oil fumes
(D) Dust particles
(E) Cigarette smoke

220. The most common asbestos-related tumor in humans is

(A) bronchogenic carcinoma
(B) carcinoma of the colon
(C) pleural mesothelioma
(D) peritoneal mesothelioma
(E) pericardial mesothelioma

221. Prolonged exposure to polyvinyl chlorides in production is associated with each of the following EXCEPT

(A) acroosteolysis
(B) Raynaud phenomenon
(C) lung disease
(D) angiosarcoma of the liver
(E) scleroderma

222. All the following statements about nonionizing radiation are true EXCEPT

(A) it includes radiowave and microwave frequencies
(B) its main adverse effects are related to thermal injury
(C) excess exposure has been associated with an increased incidence of neoplasms of the CNS
(D) excess exposure has been associated with an increased incidence of cataracts
(E) excess exposure has been associated with spermatotoxicity

223. The industry that has the highest accidental death rate in the United States is

(A) manufacturing
(B) construction
(C) mining and quarrying
(D) transportation and public utilities
(E) service

224. Rheumatologic conditions associated with occupational exposures include all the following EXCEPT

(A) Raynaud phenomenon
(B) carpal tunnel syndrome
(C) acroosteolysis
(D) systemic lupus erythematosus (SLE)
(E) gout

225. The development of mesothelioma is a dreaded consequence of exposure to asbestos. Asbestos-related mesothelioma is characterized by

(A) a lifetime incidence of about 10 percent among persons with heavy exposure to asbestos
(B) an increased incidence in smokers
(C) an incidence that does not depend upon the type of asbestos fiber
(D) a mean latency of about 10 years after exposure
(E) none of the above

226. Radiologic findings specific for exposure to asbestos include

(A) bilateral pulmonary fibrosis
(B) pulmonary nodules
(C) pleural effusion
(D) diaphragmatic calcification
(E) none of the above

227. True statements about byssinosis include which of the following?

(A) It mainly occurs in persons in the aluminum-smelting industry
(B) It mainly affects persons with hyperreactive airways
(C) It classically becomes more symptomatic later in the work week
(D) It causes bronchoconstriction and cough
(E) None of the above

228. True statements about pneumoconiosis of coal workers (black lung) include which of the following?

(A) Progressive massive fibrosis occurs in more than half of coal workers who have pneumoconiosis
(B) Inhalation of anthracite (hard coal) dust is more dangerous than inhalation of bituminous (soft coal) dust
(C) Generally, large dust particles cause more scar formation than small dust particles
(D) It is not seen with silica-free coal dust
(E) None of the above

229. Based on studies of persons who have been poisoned by chronic exposure, methyl mercury has biologic properties that include an ability to

(A) cause atrophy of the cells of the cerebellum and cerebral cortex
(B) accumulate primarily in the liver and kidneys
(C) cause restrictive lung disease
(D) be eliminated from body tissues mostly by the kidney
(E) do none of the above

230. Pneumoconiosis of coal workers (black lung) is correctly characterized by which of the following statements?

(A) Development appears to be independent of duration of exposure to coal dust
(B) Only nonsmokers are covered under the Black Lung Act
(C) It is easy to differentiate from silicosis on chest radiographs
(D) It is usually not associated with functional abnormalities of the lung
(E) None of the above

231. Workers associated with occupational exposure to lead include all the following EXCEPT

(A) battery makers
(B) painters
(C) coal miners
(D) solderers
(E) gasoline station attendants

232. Metals that have been associated with an increased incidence of lung cancer in occupationally exposed workers include

(A) copper
(B) iron
(C) chromium
(D) silver
(E) gold

233. Loss of hearing due to exposure to noise depends upon all the following factors EXCEPT

(A) the duration of exposure
(B) the intensity of noise
(C) whether the noise is continuous or intermittent
(D) the spectrum (frequency composition) of the noise
(E) the atonality of the sound

234. True statements about occupational asthma include which of the following?

(A) It accounts for about 50 percent of asthma in adults
(B) It usually improves on the weekends
(C) Diagnosis requires skin testing or serology
(D) It affects mainly persons with otherwise normal airways
(E) None of the above

235. True statements about occupational skin disease include which of the following?

(A) Most cases of contact dermatitis are mediated by an allergic reaction
(B) Allergic contact dermatitis rarely recurs upon reexposure
(C) Chloracne is usually caused by exposure to chlorine gas or hydrochloric acid
(D) A diagnostic feature of chloracne is the presence of yellowish cysts early in the disease
(E) None of the above

236. Health care workers whose fetuses or infants are at special risk include which of the following?

(A) A psychiatrist who is trying to get pregnant
(B) A pregnant dermatologist who scrubs with povidone-iodine solution
(C) An oncology nurse, in her first trimester of pregnancy, who mixes chemotherapeutic agents
(D) A breast-feeding intensive care unit nurse who wears a lead apron and is exposed to portable radiography
(E) None of the above

237. True statements about lung diseases caused by inhalation of particles of crystalline silica include all the following EXCEPT

(A) they are the most common occupational lung diseases in the world
(B) they can be seen in persons with brief but intense exposures to silica dust
(C) chest radiographs may show eggshell calcifications in hilar lymph nodes
(D) they are mediated by an immunologic reaction
(E) they are characterized by development of pulmonary nodules

238. The most prevalent mental health disorder in young children is

(A) autism
(B) mental retardation
(C) behavioral problems
(D) schizophrenia
(E) depression

239. Epidemiologic investigations of dementia have found

(A) that more than 90 percent of patients in nursing homes are demented
(B) that it is the most common cause of death among nursing home residents
(C) that more than 10 million persons in the U.S. have Alzheimer's disease
(D) that there is an increased incidence of Alzheimer's disease among relatives of patients with that disease
(E) none of the above

240. Epidemiologic studies of homosexuality have shown

(A) that the prevalence of homosexuality in the U.S. has increased in the past 20 years
(B) that homosexuality is five times as common among men as among women
(C) that the overall prevalence of homosexuality in the U.S. is about 1 percent
(D) that there is an increased incidence of homosexuality among relatives of male homosexuals
(E) none of the above

241. The most prevalent psychiatric disorder among opiate addicts undergoing treatment is

(A) schizophrenia
(B) depression
(C) alcoholism
(D) antisocial personality
(E) mania

242. Which of the following statements about the statistics of suicide is correct?

(A) Compared with other sex-race groups, the mortality from suicide is highest in black males of all ages
(B) The incidence of suicide attempts is higher in males than in females
(C) The risk of suicide increases for several months following divorce, separation, or death of the spouse
(D) Suicide rates do not correlate with socioeconomic status
(E) None of the above

243. True statements about the relationship between mental retardation and ingestion of lead in the U.S. include

(A) there are about 2 million children at risk
(B) effects on the central nervous system are reversible with chelating agents
(C) diagnosis of lead toxicity is complex
(D) mental retardation is a late consequence of toxicity
(E) none of the above

244. What proportion of the United States population is estimated to have a mental or emotional problem that requires therapy?

(A) 1 percent
(B) 5 percent
(C) 10 percent
(D) 20 percent
(E) 40 percent

245. The psychosis most likely to occur in young adults (ages 15 to 24) is

(A) schizophrenia
(B) affective psychosis
(C) involutional melancholia
(D) agitated depression
(E) none of the above

246. In most states, the legal limit for blood alcohol concentration allowed for operating a motor vehicle is

(A) 50 mg/dL
(B) 100 mg/dL
(C) 200 mg/dL
(D) 300 mg/dL
(E) 400 mg/dL

247. The highest prevalence of alcoholism is found among residents of

(A) rural areas
(B) small towns
(C) small cities
(D) the centers of large cities
(E) suburban areas of large cities

248. Which of the following statements about alcoholism is true?

(A) There are about 30 million alcoholics in the U.S.
(B) About 10 percent of the population consumes 95 percent of the alcohol
(C) The incidence of alcoholism is highest among college graduates
(D) The incidence of alcoholism is about the same in men and women
(E) None of the above

249. Studies of the epidemiology of alcoholism have shown

(A) that it is often associated with a family history of strict abstinence
(B) that there is only weak evidence for a genetic cause
(C) that the usual age of onset in men is about age 40, during the midlife crisis
(D) that there is a secondary peak in incidence after age 65
(E) none of the above

250. Which statement best represents a correct and generally accepted finding obtained in current epidemiologic studies of autistic children?

(A) Autistic children are most often members of lower socioeconomic families
(B) Autistic children are most often members of higher socioeconomic families
(C) Parents of autistic children are often emotionally frigid and introverted
(D) Autism is more prevalent among boys than girls
(E) Autism does not have a genetic cause

251. Which of the following persons is most likely to commit suicide?

(A) A 16-year-old girl
(B) A 65-year-old widower
(C) A 40-year-old married father
(D) A 30-year-old unmarried woman
(E) A 30-year-old divorced man

252. Which of the following statements best describes the incidence of suicide?

(A) The peak incidence of suicide occurs in persons who are in their early twenties and then the incidence declines
(B) The peak incidence of suicide occurs in middle-aged persons and then the incidence declines
(C) The incidence of suicide increases directly with age
(D) The incidence of suicide decreases directly with age
(E) The incidence of suicide is equal at all ages

253. Which of the following statements about the relationship between religion and suicide in the U.S. is true?

(A) There is no relationship between religion and suicide
(B) Catholics are at a higher risk of suicide than Protestants
(C) Catholics are at a higher risk of suicide than Jews
(D) Religious people are at a higher risk of suicide than those who are not religious
(E) None of the above

254. A patient presenting with new onset of mania should be questioned carefully about occupational exposures to certain chemicals, including

(A) manganese
(B) lithium
(C) cobalt
(D) aluminum
(E) none of the above

255. True statements about social determinants of health include all the following EXCEPT

(A) divorced persons have greater mortality from cancer than do married persons
(B) persons with few social ties (friends, activities) have greater mortality from coronary heart disease than do persons with many social ties
(C) persons of lower socioeconomic status have greater mortality from diabetes than do persons of higher socioeconomic status
(D) after correcting for race and access to medical care, there is still a relationship between socioeconomic status and mortality
(E) female sex is associated with increased mortality from most diseases

256. Chronic barbiturate abuse is particularly common among

(A) unemployed teen-agers
(B) college students
(C) middle-aged women
(D) elderly women
(E) elderly men

257. Which of the following mental disorders has its highest incidence in the geriatric population?

(A) Involutional depression
(B) Hysteria
(C) Obsessive-compulsive disorder
(D) Schizophrenia
(E) None of the above

258. Which of the following features characterizes families in which spouse abuse occurs?

(A) Husbands of battered women have less education than those of non-battered women
(B) Women who were abused as children are more likely to be abused by their spouses
(C) Women whose mothers suffered abuse are unlikely to be abused by their own husbands
(D) Men who batter women are prosecuted in 25 percent of cases
(E) None of the above

259. The incidence of anorexia nervosa has been increasing recently. True statements about this disease include

(A) it is two to three times more common in females than males
(B) there is an increased incidence in the middle and upper classes
(C) it usually involves a profound loss of appetite in its early stages
(D) its usual age of onset is in the twenties or thirties
(E) none of the above

260. The mental disorders that appear to be more prevalent among males include

(A) alcoholism and drug abuse
(B) schizophrenia
(C) neuroses
(D) affective disorders
(E) none of the above

261. Panic disorders are characterized by the sudden onset of overwhelming terror or anxiety. True statements about the incidence of panic disorders include which of the following?

(A) They are twice as common in women as in men
(B) The usual age of onset is less than 15 years or greater than 40 years
(C) There is an increased incidence in family members of index patients
(D) They affect about 1 in 1,000 persons
(E) None of the above

262. Which of the following statements correctly describes emotional disturbances of the postpartum period?

(A) They are more common after the birth of male children
(B) They are more common with increasing parity
(C) They rarcly last more than 1 week
(D) They occur in at least 20 percent of women
(E) None of the above

263. Parents who abuse their children are correctly characterized by all the following statements EXCEPT

(A) they are more likely to be alcoholics than are nonabusive parents
(B) they are found in all social classes
(C) they are more likely to have been abused as children than are non-abusive parents
(D) they are more likely to be men than women
(E) they are usually psychologically immature

264. True statements about the use of opioid drugs in the U.S. include

(A) the highest rates of use occur among persons 30 to 40 years of age
(B) more men than women use opioid drugs other than heroin
(C) the number of male users of heroin is 50 percent greater than the number of female users
(D) less than 1 percent of enlisted personnel in the military use opioid drugs
(E) none of the above

265. Stuttering is a disturbance of the normal speech rhythm and fluency and is characterized by

(A) an increased incidence in girls compared with boys
(B) an increased incidence among family members of stutterers
(C) an increased incidence in whites compared with nonwhites
(D) a peak incidence among adolescents
(E) none of the above

266. Studies of attempted (unsuccessful) suicide have shown which of the following?

(A) It is 100 times more common than completed (successful) suicide
(B) About 10 percent of persons who attempt suicide eventually commit suicide
(C) It is most common in persons with obsessive-compulsive personalities
(D) It is more common among women than men
(E) None of the above

267. Population-based epidemiologic surveys in the U.S. using standardized diagnostic interviews have been conducted among adults ages 18 and over. According to the responses to these surveys, which of the following statements is true?

(A) Alcohol abuse or dependence is the most prevalent mental disorder among men over age 65
(B) About one person in twenty has been affected by a significant mental disorder within the previous 6 months
(C) Most persons affected by a mental disorder are receiving some sort of psychiatric care
(D) Phobias are the most prevalent mental disorder in women of all ages
(E) None of the above

268. Persons at an increased risk of bladder cancer include workers in all the following industries EXCEPT

(A) manufacture of rubber
(B) dyeing of textiles
(C) manufacture of paint
(D) manufacture of steel
(E) printing

269. What percentage of motor vehicle fatalities are associated with drivers who are legally intoxicated?

(A) 10 percent
(B) 25 percent
(C) 50 percent
(D) 75 percent
(E) None of the above

DIRECTIONS: Each group of questions below consists of lettered headings followed by a set of numbered items. For each numbered item select the **one** lettered heading with which it is **most** closely associated. Each lettered heading may be used **once, more than once, or not at all.**

Questions 270–273

Match each of the diseases below with the pattern of occurrence in day-care centers.

(A) Infection affects children in day care, day-care center staff, and close family members
(B) Infection is generally unapparent in the children, but symptomatic in adult contacts
(C) Infection is mild in children in day care and in adult contacts, but may cause significant disease in the fetus if pregnant women are exposed
(D) Infection does not occur at an increased rate in day-care centers
(E) None of the above

270. Hepatitis A

271. Cytomegalovirus

272. Giardiasis

273. Leptospirosis

Questions 274–276

For each disease or condition, select the best available source of information.

(A) Death certificates
(B) Household surveys
(C) Cancer registry
(D) State health department
(E) Life insurance companies

274. Incidence of meningococcal meningitis in Connecticut

275. Prevalence of arthritis

276. Survival rate of patients with cancer of the pancreas

Questions 277–280

Match each group of diseases with the correct description.

(A) Bacterial infections
(B) Zoonoses
(C) Person-to-person spread
(D) Viral infections
(E) Arthropod-borne infections

277. Rabies, psittacosis, salmonellosis

278. Influenza, yellow fever, chickenpox

279. Pneumococcal, streptococcal, brucellar infections

280. Measles, shigellosis, scabies

Questions 281–284

Various terms and parameters are used in epidemiologic studies of infectious diseases. Match each statement below with the most appropriate descriptive term.

(A) Immunogenicity
(B) Pathogenicity
(C) Contagiousness
(D) Virulence
(E) None of the above

281. Neutralizing antibody develops in 95 percent of people after an attack of measles

282. Febrile respiratory tract disease develops in approximately 80 percent of children infected with influenza

283. Death occurs in approximately 20 percent of cases of pneumococcal meningitis

284. Approximately 50 percent of household contacts of a child who has a common cold become infected

Questions 285–288

Choose the most likely infectious agent for each description of the events following consumption of food.

(A) Staphylococcal enterotoxin
(B) *Clostridium botulinum* toxin
(C) Enterotoxic *Escherichia coli*
(D) *Clostridium perfringens*
(E) *Salmonella typhimurium*

285. Within 4 h after attending a church supper, 25 persons report the abrupt onset of nausea, vomiting, and abdominal cramps

286. One week after arriving in Africa, 16 students develop vomiting, severe diarrhea, and abdominal cramps lasting 2 to 3 days

287. A patient dies of respiratory failure after an illness characterized by weakness, diplopia, and cranial nerve paresis

288. One-third of the persons who attended a school banquet develop abdominal cramps and watery diarrhea 8 to 12 h later. These symptoms end within 24 h

Questions 289-292

Match each of the descriptions below with the correct type of arthritis.

(A) Gout
(B) Rheumatoid arthritis
(C) Osteoarthritis
(D) Sarcoid arthritis
(E) None of the above

289. It is often iatrogenic

290. It usually begins in childhood

291. It is the most common form of arthritis in the southeastern U.S.

292. One subtype is associated with HLA-B27

Questions 293-296

Match each of the chronic diseases below with the virus with which it has been most closely associated.

(A) Hepatitis A virus (HAV)
(B) Hepatitis B virus (HBV)
(C) Epstein-Barr virus (EBV)
(D) Adenovirus
(E) Cytomegalovirus (CMV)

293. Nasopharyngeal carcinoma

294. Hepatoma

295. Burkitt lymphoma

296. Polyarteritis nodosa

Questions 297-301

Many occupational environments contain airborne substances that cause lung disease. For each disease, select the worker with whom it is associated.

(A) Sugar cane worker
(B) Ceramic worker
(C) Arc welder
(D) Coal worker
(E) Textile worker

297. Berylliosis

298. Bagassosis

299. Byssinosis

300. Rheumatoid pneumoconiosis

301. Siderosis

Questions 302-306

Match each of the workers or hobbyists below with the infectious disease for which they are at risk.

(A) Brucellosis
(B) Hepatitis B
(C) Histoplasmosis
(D) Legionnaires' disease
(E) Sporotrichosis

302. Butchers

303. Gardeners

304. Air-conditioning workers

305. Dentists

306. Spelunkers (cave explorers)

Questions 307–311

Match each of the workers below with the factor that constitutes the principal hazard to health.

(A) Silica dust
(B) Noise
(C) Vinyl acetate
(D) Hydrogen sulfide
(E) Asbestos

307. Artist

308. Potter

309. Glass manufacturer

310. Sewer worker

311. Foundry worker

Questions 312–315

For each of the age groups below, select the most common cause of death.

(A) Heart disease
(B) Cancer
(C) Stroke
(D) Pneumonia
(E) Automobile crashes

312. 1 to 14 years

313. 15 to 24 years

314. 25 to 44 years

315. 45 to 64 years

Questions 316–320

Certain substances in the occupational environment have been identified as carcinogenic agents based on epidemiologic evidence obtained in studies of exposed laboratory animal and human populations. Match each chemical agent with the human target site for cancer.

(A) Skin
(B) Brain, liver
(C) Bladder
(D) Nasal cavities
(E) Hematopoietic system

316. β-Naphthylamine (aminonaphthalene)

317. Benzene (benzol)

318. Nickel

319. Chromium

320. Vinyl chloride

Questions 321–324

Match each substance below with the disease or condition most likely to be caused by occupational exposure.

(A) Cancer
(B) Chronic bronchitis
(C) Chronic neurologic disease
(D) Pneumoconiosis
(E) Chronic hepatitis

321. Coal

322. Methyl mercury

323. Sulfur dioxide

324. Thallium

DIRECTIONS: The group of questions below consists of four lettered headings followed by a set of numbered items. For each numbered item select

A	if the item is associated with	(A) **only**
B	if the item is associated with	(B) **only**
C	if the item is associated with	**both** (A) and (B)
D	if the item is associated with	**neither** (A) nor (B)

Each lettered heading may be used **once, more than once, or not at all.**

Questions 325–328

(A) Tobacco
(B) Alcohol
(C) Both
(D) Neither

325. Esophageal cancer

326. Cervical cancer

327. Duodenal ulcer

328. Hip fracture

Epidemiology of Health and Disease

Answers

131. **The answer is B.** *(Wilson, ed 12. pp 1016–1017.)* Hypertension, not hyper-cholesterolemia, is the major risk factor for aortic dissection. Several diseases of connective tissue—including Marfan's syndrome, Hurler's disease, and cystic medial necrosis—are associated with an increased incidence of aortic dissection. Operative mortality is about 50 percent for emergency surgery for ascending aortic dissection. Acute dissection usually presents with chest pain, classically a tearing pain that radiates to the back.

132. **The answer is C.** *(Last, ed 12. p 297.)* About 6 percent of patients admitted to general hospitals in the United States acquire an infection while in the hospital. University and municipal hospitals generally have higher rates of nosocomial infections than small community hospitals. The incidence is two to three times higher in chronic-disease hospitals compared with acute-care institutions.

133. **The answer is E.** *(Mausner, ed 2. pp 344–345.)* The most important risk factor for breast cancer (like most cancers) is age: the rate in women 75 to 84 years old is about 50 times that of women 35 to 44 years old. If crude incidence rates are compared (new cases per 100,000 adult women), one country may have much larger numbers of women in the peak risk groups and have a much higher incidence for that reason. Therefore, either comparison of the age-specific rates for each age group or else some type of *age adjustment* is essential. Although nursing may have a protective effect on breast cancer, it is of nowhere near the magnitude of the effect of age. Cigarette smoke is not a major risk factor for breast cancer. Early diagnosis, if it had any effect, would be expected to increase the incidence rate (since some cases might be discovered that otherwise might spontaneously resolve or not be noticed before the woman died of another cause). Finally, efficacy of treatment might affect the death rate, but would not affect the incidence of the disease.

134. **The answer is E.** *(Wilson, ed 12. pp 1298–1299.)* Appendicitis remains an important cause of morbidity in the Western world. Although its incidence is increasing, the mortality is decreasing. Boys and girls are about equally affected (with perhaps a 3:2 ratio of boys to girls). It is most common in the second and third decades of life. During pregnancy, displacement of the appendix by the gravid uterus can make diagnosis difficult.

135. The answer is D. *(Wegman, Pediatrics 80:817-827, 1987; 84:943-957, 1989.)* Infant mortality is defined as the number of deaths in infants up to 1 year of age per 1,000 *live* births. It is further divided into neonatal mortality, which includes deaths up to 28 days of age, and postneonatal mortality, which includes deaths from 28 days to 1 year of age. In the U.S., about two-thirds of infant mortality occurs in the first 28 days of life, and the most important cause is prematurity. The most important cause of postneonatal mortality is the sudden infant death syndrome (SIDS). American blacks have twice the rates of low birth weight, neonatal mortality, and postneonatal mortality of whites.

136. The answer is E. *(Wilson, ed 12. pp 1298-1299.)* Perforation of the appendix, with subsequent peritonitis, is the main complication of appendicitis. Up to 80 percent of infants with appendicitis will have perforated appendices at the time of presentation. Surgical mortality is 30 times higher in the presence of perforation.

137. The answer is E. *(Benenson, ed 15. pp 83-86.)* The major problems associated with chickenpox are its significant morbidity in children, including its association with Reye syndrome and the administration of aspirin; the reactivation of the virus as herpes zoster in later life; and the high morbidity and mortality in immunosuppressed patients. The case fatality rate of chickenpox in normal children is very low. Malformations from gestational chickenpox exposure are very rare (*rubella* is the disease for which this is the major concern). Infection generally confers lifelong immunity, so reinfection is rare. The *incubation* period during which time the patient is asymptomatic is up to 3 weeks, but the *prodromal* period (of mild symptoms) is short.

138. The answer is D. *(Benenson, ed 15. pp 182-185.)* Giardiasis occurs all over the world, and epidemics resulting from contamination of water supplies by the protozoan *Giardia lamblia* have occurred in Russia and the United States. Giardiasis is usually a noninvasive infection of the small intestine and has a spectrum of illness ranging from asymptomatic carriage to severe chronic diarrhea. Unlike *Entamoeba histolytica*, the cause of amebiasis, *G. lamblia* does not invade the colonic mucosa. Person-to-person transmission is frequent in day-care centers.

139. The answer is E. *(Rudolph, ed 18. p 567.)* For every infant with classic symptoms of CMV infection—including microcephaly, chorioretinitis, deafness, hepatosplenomegaly, jaundice, and thrombocytopenia—there are probably 20 infants without symptoms. Neurologic sequelae of intrauterine exposure to CMV include mental retardation, minimal cerebral dysfunction, and sensorineural hearing loss. The prevalence of infection at birth is as high as 2.5 percent in some communities.

140. The answer is B. *(Wilson, ed 12. p 1048.)* Boys develop asthma about twice as commonly as girls. Childhood asthma tends to be more allergic. There are higher levels of IgE in the serum, more frequent positive responses to inhaled antigens, and seasonal variations.

141. The answer is C. *(Rudolph, ed 18. pp 485, 1696.)* The most common causes (in decreasing order of incidence) of bacterial meningitis in children 3 months to 6 years of age are *Haemophilus influenzae* type b, *Neisseria meningitidis*, and *Streptococcus pneumoniae*. The latter two bacteria cause most cases of meningitis in adults. *Escherichia coli* K1 and group *B Streptococcus* are the most common causes of neonatal meningitis.

142. The answer is E. *(Last, ed 12. pp 301–302.)* Transmission of bacteria from patient to patient most often occurs via the hands of hospital personnel. Airborne transmission, indirect exposure, and common-source exposure do occur but are much less important than direct spread. Indwelling catheters are an important risk factor for nosocomial infection but are not sources of transmission of infections.

143. The answer is D. *(Wilson, ed 12. p 1048.)* Acute episodes of asthma have been associated with a wide variety of triggers; the exact mechanisms for many are unknown. Along with environmental allergens (such as dander or animal hair), there are chemical triggers (ozone pollution) and emotional factors. Medications, including the use of beta blockers for glaucoma, can also be responsible.

144. The answer is E. *(Trunkey, Sci Am 249:29, 1983.)* Efforts to reduce drunk driving through increased penalties, including mandatory jail terms, have been unsuccessful in the United States and Europe. Rehabilitation programs also have been unsuccessful. There is some evidence of a significant decrease in the rate of drunk driving arrests in a population when drunk driving convictions result in suspension of the driver's license.

145. The answer is D. *(Mandell, pp 388–389.)* According to surveys by the United States Centers for Disease Control, about 40 percent of all nosocomial infections involved the urinary tract. Infections of the urinary tract, surgical wounds, and the respiratory tract composed about 80 percent of all nosocomial infections. Over 85 percent of the urinary tract infections were caused by gram-negative, enteric bacteria.

146. The answer is E. *(Last, ed 12. p 1404.)* The homicide rate in the U.S. in 1980 was 10.5 per 100,000 per year, about 10 times higher than that in most Western European countries. For example, homicide rates in other countries were as follows: England and Wales 0.7, Netherlands 0.8, Iceland 0.9, France 1.0, Norway 1.1, Sweden 1.2, West Germany 1.2, Denmark 1.3, Northern Ireland, 4.2.

147. The answer is C. *(Wilson, ed 12. pp 1327-1328.)* Most cases of posttransfusion hepatitis are due to hepatitis C virus; until recently, there was no way to screen for this virus. The risk is highest for products, such as individual clotting factors, obtained from multiple pooled donors. Albumin and immune globulin convey no risk because these products receive special treatments. Hepatitis C can be a serious illness and progress to chronic hepatitis in about half of cases.

148. The answer is A. *(Last, ed 12. pp 1170-1171, 1231.)* Obesity is the major risk factor for non-insulin-dependent diabetes, but it is relatively unimportant as a risk factor for coronary heart disease, except at extremes of the weight distribution. Obesity is commonly considered to be present when body fat exceeds 25 percent of body weight in men, and 30 percent of body weight in women. Both behavioral and genetic factors contribute to obesity.

149. The answer is E. *(Wilson, ed 12. pp 1576-1577.)* Cancer is the second leading cause of death in the U.S. (after heart disease). About 500,000 Americans die annually from cancer, one-third from lung cancer. The mortality from lung cancer has been rising since at least the 1930s and has increased 50 percent in the last 15 years.

150. The answer is C. *(Last, ed 12. p 1475.)* The decayed, missing, or filled (DMF) rate is the average number of teeth per person that are identified as decayed, missing, or filled. The DMF rate is used to determine the prevalence of caries. The calculus index and the oral hygiene index measure the amount of plaque and debris formation. These indices are indirectly related to dental caries since plaque formation precedes the development of caries. The malocclusion index is a measure of the need for orthodontic care and is therefore unrelated to dental caries.

151. The answer is B. *(Rudolph, ed 18. pp 540, 577.)* Outbreaks of fever, pharyngitis, and conjunctivitis have been linked to transmission of adenovirus in swimming pools. Although the effects of penicillin on the course of pharyngitis have been debated for some time, it is now clear that resolution is hastened by penicillin, at least in children. Although rhinoviruses can be transmitted before the onset of symptoms, patients are most infectious when the symptoms are the worst. Numerous viruses, including adenovirus, herpes simplex, influenza, and parainfluenza viruses can cause sore throats, but the most common identifiable pathogen is easily the group A streptococcus, which accounts for about a third of cases.

152. The answer is D. *(Wilson, ed 12. pp 969-970.)* There is wide variation in mortality for coronary artery bypass surgery performed by different surgeons and hospitals, and this variation cannot be explained simply by differences in severity of disease. Operative mortality is also higher among the elderly. Perioperative myocardial infarction occurs in about 5 to 10 percent of patients; usually, the infarcts are small.

153.   The answer is C. *(Wilson, ed 12. pp 411-417.)* Arthritis, particularly of the hip, is more common in obese subjects, probably because of mechanical stresses on the joints. Recent studies have shown that it is not only the number of calories consumed but their composition that determines weight gain. Normal subjects can compensate for excessive carbohydrate intake by increasing their metabolic rate. Obese subjects are less active than normal subjects, but the inactivity is probably at least partially a result, rather than a cause, of the obesity. The association between hypertension and obesity is real; it is not a result of inappropriate cuff size.

154.   The answer is D. *(Rudolph, ed 18. pp 158-159, 1019-1021.)* Colostrum and mature breast milk contain and provide to infants significant amounts of immunoglobulins, especially secretory IgA. The immunoglobulins, along with other resistance factors such as maternal macrophages, contribute to the lower incidence of infections in breast-fed compared with bottle-fed infants. Infants absorb more iron from human than from bovine milk. Cow's milk may also lead to iron deficiency by increasing occult gastrointestinal blood loss.

155.   The answer is E. *(Whitney, ed 2. pp 64-67.)* Although sugar is popularly believed to be the cause of many ills, current evidence has demonstrated a causal role only for tooth decay. Like other carbohydrates, sugar is rapidly broken down to monosaccharides (glucose and fructose), so the metabolic effects are similar. Sugar is different mainly because of its sweet taste, and the fact that it is available in such pure form—unaccompanied by vitamins, minerals, or fiber. For this reason, excessive consumption of sugar may interfere with a balanced diet.

156.   The answer is E. *(Wilson, ed 12. p 995.)* In the U.S., coronary heart disease is the leading cause of death in men by age 35 and women by age 45. For unclear reasons, women are more likely to have angina (as opposed to myocardial infarction or sudden death) as their initial manifestation of coronary heart disease than are men.

157.   The answer is B. *(Last, ed 12. pp 1133-1158.)* Colon cancer accounts for about 20 percent of all cancer deaths in the U.S. It is the second leading cause of cancer death in men (after lung cancer) and the third leading cause of cancer death in women (after lung and breast cancer). The cause is unknown but may be related to the action of certain components of the diet, such as saturated fats, on the colonic mucosa.

158.   The answer is A. *(Wilson, ed 12. pp 1019-1020.)* The majority of patients with peripheral vascular disease (the usual cause of intermittent claudication) also have coronary artery disease; the opposite is not true. Risk factors for the two types of vascular disease (peripheral and coronary) appear to be similar. Only about 5 percent of patients with intermittent claudication eventually require amputation.

159. The answer is A. *(Wilson, ed 12. pp 1249-1250.)* The incidence of gastric cancer in men is twice that in women. Gastric cancer is common in Japan, Chile, and in parts of Eastern Europe and is much less common in the United States. The steady decline in the incidence of gastric cancer in the United States over the past 40 years has not been adequately explained. Japanese people who have migrated to the United States continue to have a high incidence, but the incidence in their offspring tends more toward the general incidence of the United States. These data are evidence of an environmental etiologic factor in the disease. Also, some evidence has been obtained for a genetic factor: gastric cancer is two to four times more common in relatives of persons who have this disease than in relatives of persons who do not have this disease. Smokers and patients with benign gastric ulcers are not at increased risk.

160. The answer is E. *(Wyngaarden, ed 18. p 35.)* Because they affect young people disproportionately, injuries are the most important cause of premature loss of life in the U.S. Cancer, which also has a relatively high incidence among the young, is second. Coronary disease, the most important overall cause of death, mainly affects older persons. Congenital heart disease is too rare to be an important cause of premature loss of life. In some communities, AIDS is now the leading cause of premature loss of life.

161. The answer is E. *(Last, ed 12. pp 1297-1311.)* Chronic infection of the tarsal conjunctiva with *Chlamydia trachomatis* causes blindness by scarring of the eyelids and eventual opacification of the exposed cornea, not by predisposing to retinal detachment. The poorer the hygiene, the greater the chance for reinfection; thus trachoma is the leading cause of blindness among persons who live in dry environments without access to sufficient water for washing. Cataracts are also a common cause of blindness in the third world because of inadequate access to surgical facilities. In the U.S., the leading cause of blindness among whites is retinal disease, especially senile macular degeneration; among blacks, glaucoma is the most important (and preventable) cause. Persons with high degrees of myopia (nearsightedness) have elongated eyes, with thin retinas that are susceptible to detachment. Type I (and, to a lesser extent, type II) diabetics are at risk for proliferative retinopathy. In this condition, new blood vessels form on the retina; these vessels are fragile and may cause vitreous hemorrhage and retinal detachment.

162. The answer is D. *(Wilson, ed 12. p 1526.)* Cobalamin deficiency can be caused by a variety of conditions. Some are due to the development of auto-immunity and thus have an increased incidence in patients with a personal or family history of autoimmune disorders, such as Graves' disease or pernicious anemia. Others are due to malabsorption or to the destruction of the gastric parietal cells that produce intrinsic factor, which can be seen following gastric injury. Infection with the fish tapeworm (*Diphyllobothrium latum*) can also cause B_{12} deficiency; this parasite is a cestode, not a nematode.

163.   The answer is B. *(Wilson, ed 12. pp 1520-1521.)* The most common causes of microcytic anemia in the U.S. are iron deficiency, lead poisoning, thalassemia, and the anemia of chronic disease. Iron deficiency on a dietary basis is the most common cause in children and menstruating or pregnant women. However, iron deficiency is rarely seen on a dietary basis in men; finding it mandates a search for a (gastrointestinal) site of blood loss. Pica (a desire to eat unusual substances) can be a cause of microcytic anemia if it involves eating lead paint chips; sometimes pica (e.g., a desire to eat ice) is even seen as a manifestation of iron deficiency. Although the iron in breast milk is highly bioavailable, it is insufficient to keep pace with growth beyond the first 4 to 6 months of life; breast-fed babies thus require an additional iron source (such as fortified cereal) at that time.

164.   The answer is A. *(Wilson, ed 12. p 1293.)* Prognosis in colon cancer depends upon a variety of factors, including some related to the characteristics of the cancer cells, others to the stage of the disease. Other prognostic factors may include specific patterns of chromosomal deletions. When adjusted for these other factors, tumor size is not an independent predictor of poor outcome.

165.   The answer is C. *(Last, ed 12. pp 1225-1239.)* The prevalence of diabetes increases substantially with age, and most elderly diabetics have type II diabetes. About 2 percent of all Americans have diabetes; of those over age 70 years, the prevalence is about 10 percent. Because type II diabetes can be relatively asymptomatic, up to half of all diabetics may be undiagnosed.

166.   The answer is A. *(Wilson, ed 12. p 1437.)* Rheumatoid arthritis afflicts women three times more than men. Its highest incidence is in the fourth and fifth decades of life. Differences in race, geographic residence, and social, economic, or cultural characteristics have not been related to the prevalence of this systemic disease of unknown cause.

167.   The answer is B. *(Wilson, ed 12. p 1289.)* Evidence from international studies suggests that colon cancer rates are high in countries in which average consumption of animal fats is high. Several conditions associated with chronic inflammation of the colon—including Crohn's disease, ulcerative colitis, and the presence of a ureterosigmoidostomy—also predispose to colon cancer. Additional risk factors may include diets low in dietary fiber.

168.   The answer is D. *(Wilson, ed 12. pp 938-952.)* Although rheumatic heart disease is still a major problem in many developing countries, its incidence in the U.S. has been declining for many years. Persons with a history of rheumatic fever are at a substantially increased risk of recurrence, and prophylactic therapy (such as monthly injections of benzathine penicillin) is recommended. Coronary artery disease does not cause any form of valvular heart disease, though it may cause mitral regurgitation with a normal valve because of papillary muscle necrosis. Echocardiographic surveys have found that up to 7 percent of women between the ages of 14 and 30 have mitral valve prolapse; most are asymptomatic.

169.   The answer is D. *(Last, ed 12. p 1242.)* Cystic fibrosis is the most common genetic disease in whites in the U.S. (sickle cell anemia is the most common genetic disease in blacks). The incidence is about 1 in 2,000 births; about 5 percent of the white population are carriers of the gene (heterozygotes). The diagnosis can be confirmed by finding elevated levels of chloride (> 60 meq/L) in the sweat. Despite suffering from severe obstructive pulmonary disease, as well as other problems like pancreatic insufficiency, about half of the patients with cystic fibrosis survive beyond age 15.

170.   The answer is D. *(Wilson, ed 12. pp 1047-1048.)* Asthma is characterized by reversible bronchospasm. Between episodes FEV_1 may be entirely normal. Its cause is unknown but may be related to intrinsic (stress) or extrinsic (allergies) factors. Pulmonary infections in infancy, especially bronchiolitis due to respiratory syncytial virus, are a major risk factor. Almost 20 percent of patients have their first attack *after* age 40. Although the disease is more frequent in boys than girls, the sex difference disappears in adulthood.

171.   The answer is B. *(Wilson, ed 12. p 1072.)* Cystic fibrosis is the most common genetic disorder in white Americans, nearly 1 in 20 of whom carries the gene. Median survival is now about 20 years. Nearly all (98 percent) men with cystic fibrosis are infertile.

172.   The answer is C. *(Wilson, ed 12. pp 1074-1078.)* The accepted diagnosis of emphysema requires examination of lung tissue. Along with chronic bronchitis, emphysema causes chronic (irreversible) obstructive airways disease; the two diseases cause similar changes in expiratory flow rates. Smokers are at least ten times more likely to develop emphysema than nonsmokers, and heavy smokers are more likely to do so than light smokers. Inhalation of coal dust is associated with pneumoconiosis, a form of restrictive lung disease.

173.   The answer is B. *(Wilson, ed 12. pp 1792-1793.)* Among women ages 40 to 44, the highest mortality occurs among those using birth control pills, especially among smokers. In general, the risks of birth control pills are about five times higher in smokers. Mortality in IUD users is similar at all ages. The highest birth-related death rates (about 28 per 100,000 women per year) occur in women ages 40 to 44; this compares with a mortality of 1.1 per 100,000 women per year associated with abortions.

174.   The answer is E. *(Last, ed 12. pp 1277–1279.)* Disorders of the musculo-skeletal system are the most common cause of limitation of activity in the U.S., affecting about 12 million persons (about 8 million persons are affected by cardiovascular disease, the second leading cause). Back and spine impairments are the most common type, accounting for about half of these cases. Persons who engage in heavy labor, especially if it involves lifting and stooping, are 50 percent more likely to have back pain than are sedentary workers. X-rays and medical examinations are not reliable ways to identify persons at high risk of sustaining a back injury; strength testing seems to be a better method.

175.   The answer is B. *(Wilson, ed 12. pp 1069–1070.)* Bronchiectasis is quite common in childhood and either may begin as an infection of the bronchi and bronchioles that causes necrosis or may be the consequence of some abnormal physiologic mechanism that causes abnormal dilatation, poor drainage, and secondary infection. Cough, fever, and production of copious amounts of malodorous sputum are characteristic symptoms of bronchiectasis, which can affect persons of any age or sex. Bronchiectasis may persist as a chronic, smoldering, latent infection.

176.   The answer is E. *(Wilson, ed 12. p 312.)* Antibiotics, especially penicillins and sulfa drugs, are the most common causes of drug reactions. Cutaneous reactions are most common and usually occur less than 1 week after exposure. Exanthem is the most common skin manifestation. The incidence of cutaneous drug reactions is not higher in the elderly.

177.   The answer is D. *(Last, ed 12. pp 1159–1163.)* The death rate due to coronary artery disease (CAD) varies greatly from country to country, from a low of about 120 per 100,000 men aged 35 to 74 years in Japan, to a high of nearly 900 per 100,000 men in Finland. Several areas of Europe (Finland, Northern Ireland, and Scotland) have higher rates than the U.S. Finland has the highest death rate due to CAD in the world; this is perhaps related to a high per capita consumption of animal fat. The low rate of CAD in Japan (one-sixth that in the U.S.) is thought to be related to diet. The death rate due to CAD has been declining about 2 percent each year since 1968 in the U.S., the most rapid decline in the world.

178.   The answer is D. *(Wilson, ed 12. p 1978.)* Transient ischemic attacks are a relatively late manifestation of cerebrovascular atherosclerosis. A patient with a transient ischemic attack has about a 6 percent chance of having stroke within

1 year, much higher than that seen in asymptomatic persons who have one or more of the *risk factors* for stroke. These risk factors include the presence of a carotid bruit, age, hypercholesterolemia, smoking, and especially hypertension. Embolic stroke is a rare complication of mitral valve prolapse but is commonly seen in persons with atrial fibrillation.

179.   The answer is E. *(Wilson, ed 12. p 16.)* Most of the differences in life expectancy between men and women are thought to be a result of lower rates of smoking, drinking of alcohol, and violent deaths in women. Nearly three times as many elderly women as men live alone; women commonly outlive their husbands. Woman are also more likely to be institutionalized, for similar reasons. In the next 40 years, the number of elderly persons in the U.S. is expected to double.

180.   The answer is C. *(Wilson, ed 12. pp 1359–1360.)* Gallstones are extremely common; about 20 percent of women over the age of 40 have them. Although most gallstones contain cholesterol, elevated levels of plasma cholesterol are *not* associated with an increased risk. Not only are diabetics at an increased risk of developing gallstones, they also have an increased morbidity and mortality associated with the disease. Chronic hemolytic anemia predisposes to the formation of calcium bilirubinate gallstones, which are more common in Asia. Additional risk factors for gallstones include age, obesity, and chronic biliary infection.

181.   The answer is C. *(Wyngaarden, ed 18. p 2012.)* Although systemic lupus erythematosus (SLE) is predominantly a disease of young women, it is much less common than rheumatoid arthritis in this age group. The female:male ratio is about 10:1. The black:white ratio is about 3:1 in the U.S. A black woman in the U.S. has about a 1 in 250 chance of developing lupus in her lifetime. Diagnosis is based on fulfilling at least 4 out of 11 criteria (such as the presence of pleurisy or pericarditis) but does not require a positive ANA test.

182.   The answer is B. *(Wilson, ed 12. p 1526.)* Folate deficiency can occur because of insufficient intake in the diet, because of malabsorption, or because of increased needs for the vitamin. Folate is found in green, leafy vegetables; strict vegetarians are at risk of deficiency of cobalamin (vitamin B_{12}), which is found in meats. Persons with chronic hemolysis, such as those with sickle cell anemia, can have increased needs for folate. Dialysis increases the need for the water-soluble (and dialyzable) vitamins.

183.   The answer is E. *(Wyngaarden, ed 18. p 576.)* Chronic renal failure is associated with accelerated atherogenesis; dialysis does not appear to slow this process. Overall mortality for patients on dialysis is approximately 5 percent per year. Depression is common. Infections with *Staphylococcus aureus*, mycobacteria, and hepatitis B have an increased incidence.

184.   The answer is D. *(Wilson, ed 12. p 147.)* Age is by far the most important risk factor for developing cataracts. Both types of diabetes are complicated by early cataract formation, possibly owing to the effect of hyperglycemia on the lens proteins. Other causes include trauma, ultraviolet radiation, and several congenital infections, such as rubella. Exposure to video display terminals causes fatigue and eye strain, much like studying for examinations.

185.   The answer is E. *(Wilson, ed 12. pp 1505-1507.)* There are two types of hemophilia: type A, or factor VIII deficiency; and type B, or factor IX deficiency. Both are sex-linked genetic disorders, which indicates that the faulty genes are carried on the X chromosome. Thus, there is no association with environmental factors or with HLA type (which is carried on chromosome 6).

186.   The answer is A. *(Wilson, ed 12. p 1577.)* In the past 25 years, age-adjusted mortality has increased for certain forms of cancer, including cancer of the lung and pancreas, probably because of cigarette smoking. The mortality of uterine cancer has declined by about 60 percent in that time, mainly owing to increased acceptance and use of the Pap test. Mortality from stomach cancer has also declined by 60 percent; the reason is unknown.

187.   The answer is A. *(Wilson, ed 12. pp 1350-1351.)* Hepatoma accounts for only 1 to 2 percent of cancers in the Western world. But in parts of the world where chronic, lifelong carriage of the hepatitis B surface antigen (HBsAg) is common, such as Africa, hepatoma is the most common cause of death from cancer in adult men and accounts for up to 40 percent of cancer deaths. In the Western world, the tumor is more commonly seen in persons with cirrhosis.

188.   The answer is D. *(Wilson, ed 12. pp 682-683.)* Recent studies have shown that infection with HSV-1 is more common and tends to occur earlier in life than infection with HSV-2. Either type of virus can cause oral or genital lesions, but genital HSV-2 infection is eight to ten times more likely to reactivate than genital HSV-1 infection. Previous infection with one type of HSV does not provide protection against subsequent infection with the other type. Reports of HSV-2 infection are twice as common using seroepidemiologic techniques as they are by clinical history.

189.   The answer is E. *(Wilson, ed 12. pp 1579-1580.)* A higher-than-normal incidence of breast, cervical, colon, and stomach cancers has been demonstrated in relatives of patients with these cancers. There are certain inherited syndromes (such as Gardner syndrome) associated with a markedly increased risk of colon cancer (nearly 100 percent). A woman who has a first-degree relative (mother, sister, daughter) with breast cancer has a threefold increased risk of developing the disease. Laryngeal cancer is related to smoking and alcohol use.

190.   The answer is E. *(Last, ed 12. pp 1149-1150.)* The relationship that exists between marital status and cancer of the cervix may be due to the increased sexual activity that usually accompanies marriage and increased exposure to possible carcinogenic agents. This theory is supported by the fact that prostitutes as well as married women have an increased frequency of cancer of the cervix. Endocrine factors may account for the difference in the risk of breast cancer between single and married women; breast cancer is more common among nulliparous women than among women who have borne children. Risk of ovarian cancer is also higher in nulliparous women.

191.   The answer is D. *(Wilson, ed 12. p 1102.)* Probably because rates of cigarette smoking in men are lower than they were 20 to 30 years ago, incidence rates of lung cancer are actually on the decline in men. However, smoking rates in women were increasing, at least until very recently, and thus rates of lung cancer continue to rise in women. Lung cancer has replaced breast cancer as the leading cause of cancer death in women.

192.   The answer is E. *(Wilson, ed 12. pp 1580-1581.)* Tobacco-related cancers (mainly lung cancer) cause more than 30 percent of all cancer deaths in the U.S. Smoking cigarettes increases the risk of lung cancer at least tenfold. As more women with a long-term smoking history enter the age with the highest incidence rate for lung cancer, rates of tobacco-related cancer among women are increasing. Pancreatic cancer is at least twice as common in smokers; smoking is a risk factor for cancer of the bladder and kidney; and oral, laryngeal, and esophageal cancers are also increased by cigarette smoke, particularly among heavy alcohol drinkers.

193.   The answer is E. *(Wilson, ed 12. pp 2039-2040.)* Although the cause of multiple sclerosis is unknown, its epidemiology has been well studied. Women compose about 60 percent of the cases. In general, the incidence of the disease increases with distance from the equator: the disease is twice as frequent in the northern as in the southern U.S. Certain HLA types, such as B7 in whites and DW2 in blacks, are more common among patients with the disease. First-degree relatives (siblings, parents) of patients with MS have an eightfold increased risk of developing the disease compared with the general population.

194.   The answer is A. *(Wilson, ed 12. p 556.)* While the majority of patients with pneumococcal pneumonia can be cured with appropriate antibiotic therapy, there are several characteristics associated with poor survival. These include patients at extremes of age (either very young or old), underlying conditions (such as alcoholism), and multilobar disease. Leukopenia, but not leukocytosis, is also associated with decreased survival.

195.   The answer is B. *(Last, ed 12. pp 1136–1137.)* The incidence of cancer of the stomach and uterine cervix has been decreasing worldwide. However, the incidence of leukemia and cancers of the lung, breast, uterine corpus, and prostate are increasing. The decrease in the incidence of cervical cancer has been attributed to use of the Pap smear; the decrease in stomach cancer has not been adequately explained.

196.   The answer is B. *(Wilson, ed 12. pp 1580, 1633.)* Exposure to ultraviolet light is generally accepted to be a cause of skin cancer. Both squamous and basal cell tumors can result from chronic exposure. Although skin cancer (not including melanoma) is by far the most common form of cancer, very few patients with skin cancer (about 1 percent) die of the disease.

197.   The answer is E. *(Wilson, ed 12. pp 1384–1385.)* Of 100 patients who have cancer of the pancreas, only one to two patients can be expected to survive 5 years after diagnosis. Early diagnosis is difficult. Patients may complain of vague abdominal pain or weakness. Tumors of the body and tail of the pancreas are rarely detected before metastases. About 15 to 20 percent of patients who have tumors of the head of the pancreas are surgical candidates for resection. Radiotherapy and chemotherapy do not prolong life.

198.   The answer is A. *(Wilson, ed 12. pp 1629–1631.)* Nearly 90 percent of men have benign prostatic hypertrophy by age 70. Prostate cancer follows cancer of the lung and cancer of the colon as a cause of cancer death in the U.S. in men. The reason the incidence of prostate cancer is about twice as high in blacks as in whites is not known.

199.   The answer is E. *(Wilson, ed 12. p 1090.)* Conditions and periods associated with a high risk of thromboembolism include the postoperative period, use of oral contraceptives, congestive heart failure, the postpartum period, chronic pulmonary disease, fractures or other injuries of lower extremities, obesity, deep venous insufficiency in the legs, prolonged bed rest, and carcinoma.

200.   The answer is C. *(Wilson, ed 12. p 1437.)* The incidence of rheumatoid arthritis is about three times higher in women than in men. Rheumatoid arthritis is nearly four times more common in first-degree relatives of cases, and there is an association with HLA-DR4. Joint destruction is a hallmark of the disease and progresses in most cases. About 80 percent of patients develop evidence of joint destruction after 10 years.

201.   The answer is D. *(Wilson, ed 12. p 1475.)* The prevalence of osteoarthritis is similar by sex, although it is slightly more common in men under the age of 45 years and among women over the age of 55 years. Osteoarthritis is almost universal by age 75. While it afflicts all races, the pattern of joint involvement varies. Heberden's nodes (swellings of the distal interphalangeal joints) are inherited in an autosomal dominant fashion.

202.   The answer is C. *(Wilson, ed 12. pp 1977-2002.)* The major risk factors for stroke are hypertension, diabetes, electrocardiographic evidence of an enlarged heart, hypercholesterolemia, and cigarette smoking. The risk increases when one of the factors is present and is further increased if more than one factor is present. There is no evidence that alcoholism is related to increased risk of stroke; and type A personality, although possibly associated with an increased risk of myocardial infarction, has not been related to an increased risk of stroke.

203.   The answer is E. *(Wilson, ed 12. pp 1439-1440.)* The course of rheumatoid arthritis is unpredictable but is worse in patients who have certain characteristics, including advanced age. White women are more likely to have progressively worsening disease than are white men. Certain serologic markers, including high titers of rheumatoid factor and high serum haptoglobin levels, are also associated with poor prognosis. Most of the progression appears to occur in the first 6 years of the disease's course. There is no relationship with the initial pattern of arthritis.

204.   The answer is D. *(Wilson, ed 12. pp 1790-1792.)* The only well-established hazard related to use of oral contraceptives is increased risk of thromboembolism. Of the changes that occur with the use of oral contraceptives, most are reversible when the drug is discontinued. There is no association between use of oral contraceptives and breast cancer or osteoporosis. The synthetic estrogen diethylstilbestrol (DES) was identified as a transplacental carcinogen: some daughters of women given the drug during pregnancy to prevent miscarriage subsequently developed adenocarcinoma of the vagina and cervix. However, DES is *not* an oral contraceptive.

205.   The answer is E. *(Wilson, ed 12. pp 1742-1743.)* Factors that predispose an adult to diabetes mellitus include increased age, familial inheritance, pregnancy, and obesity; the last is considered the most important factor. About 80 percent of adults who have maturity-onset diabetes are obese. Although the precise mode of inheritance is unknown, the genetic association is clear. A person who is over 40 years of age and who has a parent with diabetes has two to four times the risk of developing the disease. For some unknown reason, the risk is greater if the father rather than the mother has diabetes. Overt diabetes may be precipitated by pregnancy.

206.   The answer is C. *(Wilson, ed 12. pp 1074-1082.)* Contributing etiologic factors in chronic bronchitis include air pollution, occupation, infection, smoking, and genotype. Chronic bronchitis is more prevalent in urban regions where air is often polluted. Workers exposed to dusts and some gases have a higher incidence of the disease. Not only is cigarette smoking the most common single etiologic factor, it also potentiates every other factor. It impairs ciliary motility, inhibits fixation of alveolar macrophages, leads to hypertrophy of the glands, and probably causes polymorphonuclear cells to release proteolytic enzymes.

207. The answer is B. *(Wilson, ed 12. p 1971.)* About 2 to 5 percent of children will have a seizure associated with a febrile illness. Fever, trauma, and infections are the most commonly identified causes of seizures in children. Seizures are more likely with slowly growing malignancies. About half of patients with posttraumatic seizures will spontaneously recover.

208. The answer is B. *(Wilson, ed 12. pp 1753-1756.)* Diabetes is the most common cause of blindness in adults up to age 70 in the U.S. More than half of all nontraumatic amputations occur in diabetic persons with nonhealing limb ulcers or gangrene. Other complications include renal failure, coronary artery disease, and stroke. The average life expectancy of a type I (insulin-dependent) diabetic is about 20 years shorter than that of a person without diabetes.

209. The answer is B. *(Wilson, ed 12. p 1626.)* Testicular cancer is one of the most common malignancies in men between the ages of 20 and 35, when the incidence of the disease peaks; it is uncommon after the age of 40. It is more common in whites than in blacks. Males with intraabdominal testes are at several-fold increased risk. About 6,000 males develop the disease each year in the U.S.

210. The answer is A. *(Wilson, ed 12. pp 1063, 2160-2161.)* Passive, or second-hand, exposure to cigarette smoke may lead to increased levels of carbon monoxide. Children born to parents who smoke cigarettes are more likely to develop bronchiolitis and pneumonia in the first year of life than infants of nonsmoking parents. Other exposed nonsmokers may develop conjunctivitis, headache, nasal congestion, and cough. Exposure to cigarette smoke may exacerbate the symptoms of persons with chronic obstructive pulmonary disease (COPD) and angina pectoris. The incidence of lung cancer appears to be increased in nonsmoking persons married to persons who smoke compared with those married to nonsmokers.

211. The answer is E. *(Wyngaarden, ed 18. pp 1014-1022.)* Prognosis of Hodgkin's disease correlates with the stage of the disease at diagnosis. However, weight loss, fever, and chills are usually regarded as unfavorable prognostic signs and symptoms. Histologic types have been associated with their 5-year survival data: patients with the lymphocyte-predominant type have a better survival than those with the other types. Women have a better prognosis than men; the reason is unknown.

212. The answer is E. *(Wilson, ed 12. pp 1326-1327.)* Any worker whose job requires frequent contact with blood is at increased risk of exposure to hepatitis B virus. The lifetime risk to such workers is estimated to be between 15 and 30 percent compared with about 5 percent in the general population. Included are dialysis staff, oral surgeons, staff of custodial institutions, and surgeons as well as many nurses in high risk units, blood bank workers, and laboratory technicians.

213.   The answer is C. *(Wilson, ed 12. p 1269.)* Both ulcerative colitis and Crohn's disease are rare; thus, the odds ratio is a valid estimator of the relative risk. Because nearly 90 percent of Americans are white, disease rates in whites will be approximately those seen in the overall population; with a relative risk of 2.0, rates in blacks will be about half of the overall rates. Prevalence is approximately equal to incidence times the duration of disease; the diseases have a similar duration of about 15 years. With a prevalence of 100 per 100,000, there are about 240,000 persons with ulcerative colitis in the U.S. (total population of about 240 million).

214.   The answer is B. *(Raffle, p 299. Rosenstock, pp 52–57.)* Before exposure to benzene was regulated by federal statute in 1950, it was associated with a dose-dependent incidence of aplastic anemia. Exposure to benzene has also been associated with all the leukemias (with the possible exception of chronic lymphocytic leukemia). There are no clear occupational causes of non-Hodgkin lymphomas.

215.   The answer is D. *(Wilson, ed 12. pp 1527, 2101, 2185.)* Exposure to organic mercury can cause an intention tremor, or even delirium (use of mercury in the manufacture of felt hats led to the phrase "mad as a hatter"). Lead poisoning in adults causes peripheral neuropathy and ataxia; in children it can cause irreversible defects in the central nervous system. Long-term exposure to nitrous oxide (usually as a result of abuse) has been reported to cause a neuropathy similar to that seen in pernicious anemia. Exposure to arsenic can cause delirium or even coma. Exposure to sulfur dioxide mainly causes irritation of the mucous membranes.

216.   The answer is C. *(Wilson, ed 12. p 1058.)* Mesothelioma, a cancer that develops from the mesothelial cells that cover the pleural and other serous membranes, occurs almost exclusively among persons who through occupation have been chronically exposed to air containing large numbers of asbestos particles. (Pericardial mesothelioma is not associated with asbestos exposure.) Asbestos particles, each measuring 50 μm in length and 0.5 μm in diameter, generally are regarded as a causative agent for the formation of a granuloma and for the thickening of the parietal and visceral pleurae. Cancers of the bronchus and the larynx are associated with cigarette smoking. Byssinosis is a pneumoconiosis due to chronic inhalation of textile dusts.

217.   The answer is A. *(Rosenstock, pp 80–90.)* Ethylene glycol, found in antifreeze, causes an acute tubular necrosis usually seen in attempted overdoses. Chronic exposure to cadmium or lead—both of which are used in welding, soldering, and jewelry-making—causes injury to the proximal tubules and may lead to chronic renal failure; acute overexposure has been associated with oliguric renal failure. Halogenated hydrocarbons, such as carbon tetrachloride, cause acute tubular necrosis, especially if exposure is via inhalation. β-Naphthylamine, used in the rubber and dye industries, is associated with bladder cancer.

218. The answer is E. *(Wilson, ed 12. p 1633.)* More workers are exposed to sunlight than to any of the other carcinogens listed in the question. In occupations related to agriculture, construction, fishing, forestry, gardening, landscaping, road building, and telephone and electric line installation, large numbers of workers are exposed to ultraviolet light. The photosensitizing effects of certain industrial irritants and photosensitizing chemicals such as coal tar or creosols are enhanced by the ultraviolet light of the sun, so that even a short exposure in the late afternoon is likely to produce severe sunburn.

219. The answer is D. *(Wilson, ed 12. pp 1056–1060.)* Pneumoconiosis, a condition in which lung tissue reacts to permanently deposited dust particles, usually occurs as a result of occupational exposure to air containing particulate matter. Anthracosis, silicosis, asbestosis, berylliosis, farmer's lung, and byssinosis are among the more than 30 forms of pneumoconioses that have been described in the literature. Pneumoconiosis usually causes a restrictive lung disease. Sulfur oxides, nitrogen oxides, oil fumes, and cigarette smoke are likely to cause acute bronchospasm or to exacerbate preexisting diseases such as chronic bronchitis and emphysema.

220. The answer is A. *(Rosenstock, p 42.)* Mesotheliomas of the pleural and peritoneal surfaces are the classic asbestos-related tumors because they are rarely seen in persons never exposed to asbestos. However, it is important to realize that persons with exposure to asbestos are also at a tenfold increased risk of bronchogenic cancer and that this tumor is far more common than mesothelioma. Persons with extensive fibrosis due to asbestosis may have up to a 50 percent risk of developing bronchogenic cancer.

221. The answer is C. *(Last, ed 12. pp 631–632.)* Neither polyvinyl chloride (PVC) nor the vinyl chloride monomer from which it is derived have been clearly shown to cause lung disease. PVC exposure causes bone abnormalities (resorption of the distal phalanges with spontaneous fractures) called acroosteolysis. PVC can also cause a nonmalignant form of liver disease with associated portal hypertension.

222. The answer is C. *(Rosenstock, pp 185–186.)* Nonionizing radiation does not cause molecular ionization or disruption of atomic nuclei. It includes radiowaves, microwaves, and infrared, visible, and ultraviolet light. Heating of susceptible tissues causes the main harmful effects, such as skin burns and cataracts. Spermatogenesis is also adversely affected by the higher temperatures. No increase in neoplasms, with the important exception of dermatologic malignancies, has been documented.

223.   The answer is C. *(Last, ed 12. pp 1565-1566.)* Mining and quarrying is the most dangerous industry in the United States. Agriculture is second; about 50 deaths per 100,000 workers occur each year. According to recent estimates, about 109 million disabling injuries and 11,000 deaths occur annually in industrial occupations.

224.   The answer is D. *(Rosenstock, pp 61-71.)* Occupational exposures have been associated with a wide variety of rheumatologic syndromes. Some, such as Raynaud phenomenon and carpal tunnel syndrome, are thought to be caused by mechanical problems, including vibration and overuse. Others are associated with specific toxicities, such as lead-induced gout and polyvinyl chloride–induced acroosteolysis. The latter condition closely resembles scleroderma.

225.   The answer is A. *(Raffle, pp 680-683. Rosenstock, p 41.)* The mean latency period from exposure to the development of mesothelioma is 35 years. The disease often develops in the absence of radiographic asbestosis. There are no other known risk factors besides exposure to asbestos. The chrysotile type of asbestos appears to present less risk than other types.

226.   The answer is D. *(Wilson, ed 12. p 1058.)* A common finding in people who have been exposed chronically to asbestos is calcification of the pleura and dia-phragm. The pleural calcification is often unilateral. The pattern of calcification is unique and easily differentiated from that caused by trauma and surgery. Calcifica-tion of the diaphragm is so rare that this finding is almost pathognomonic for asbestosis. Bilateral fibrosis is not a specific finding in the diagnosis of asbestosis. Although pleural effusion is not specific, its presence in a patient with asbestosis should prompt a search for bronchogenic carcinoma or mesothelioma.

227.   The answer is D. *(Raffle, pp 690-705. Rosenstock, p 25.)* Byssinosis, which is derived from the Greek word for *flax*, afflicts persons who work with dusts from certain plants, such as cotton bracts, hemp, and flax. It causes bronchoconstriction, even in persons who do not have hyperreactive airways. The symptoms of byssinosis tend to be most severe when workers return after a weekend. The first description of the symptom pattern, in 1845, noted, "All the workers told us that the dust bothered them much less on the last days of the week than on Monday and Tuesday. The masters find the cause of this increased sensitivity to be in the excesses of Sun-day...." The pathophysiologic explanation for the disease is not known.

228.   The answer is B. *(Last, ed 12. pp 545-552.)* Usually, pneumoconiosis develops in coal workers who have been exposed for 10 to 20 years to coal dust that varies in size from 0.5 to 5 μm. This condition was noted to occur even in coal workers exposed to dust virtually free of silica. Anthracite dust is more dangerous for two reasons: (1) the smaller particle size causes more extensive scar formation; and (2) anthracite deposits are associated with higher levels of silica dust. Progressive massive fibrosis occurs in only a small minority of cases.

229. The answer is A. *(Last, ed 12. pp 603–606.)* Differences in the biologic properties of inorganic and organic compounds of mercury have been learned through studies in Japan, Sweden, Iraq, and Pakistan—countries where many people accidentally have been poisoned by aryl, alkyl, and alkoxyalkyl mercury compounds. In contrast to inorganic forms of mercury, which accumulate in and damage the liver and kidneys, methyl mercury collects in nervous system tissue and causes mild to severe neurologic disorders due to atrophy of cells of the cerebellum and cerebral cortex. Nearly 90 percent of ingested methyl mercury is eliminated by action of the gastrointestinal system. The mutagenicity of methyl mercury has been demonstrated both in laboratory experiments using fruit flies and in evaluation of biopsies of persons exposed to very low levels of this compound.

230. The answer is D. *(Raffle, pp 663–669. Rosenstock, p 35.)* Fortunately, pneumoconiosis is usually a mild disease and characteristically develops after 20 or more years to exposure to coal dust. Development of progressive massive fibrosis (PMF), a disabling and often fatal complication, is uncommon. Pneumoconiosis of coal workers cannot be differentiated either clinically or radiographically from silicosis; both disorders are often present in the same patient.

231. The answer is C. *(Raffle, pp 240–250. Rosenstock, pp 206–207.)* It is important to distinguish between exposures to organic and inorganic lead because they cause different syndromes. Acutely, overexposure to inorganic lead causes abdominal colic and hemolytic anemia; chronically, it causes an insidious illness characterized by fatigue, depression, and a motor neuropathy. Overexposure to organic lead causes a syndrome limited to the central nervous system, with insomnia, anorexia, irritability, and, eventually, an agitated encephalopathy. It is usually seen in workers who have been cleaning gasoline storage tanks. Gasoline station attendants are exposed to an organic lead compound, tetraethyl lead (TEL), used as an antiknock ingredient in gasolines, although they rarely develop symptoms of toxicity from this exposure.

232. The answer is C. *(Rosenstock, pp 42–43.)* Occupational exposure to several metals, including arsenic, nickel, and chromium, has been associated with lung cancer. Other occupationally encountered substances associated with lung cancer include asbestos, uranium, and coal tar pitch. There are no known cancers associated with occupational exposure to iron, silver, or gold.

233.   The answer is E. *(Last, ed 12. pp 750–757.)* A sudden loud noise can cause a punctured eardrum, which may result in a hearing loss of 20 or more decibels if the puncture is large enough. Continuous noise can cause about twice the amount of hearing loss as intermittent sound, since intermittent sound allows the hearing functions some opportunity to recover. The greatest loss of hearing occurs in the first hour of exposure and then levels off. The spectrum of the noise is also important: at the same intensity, low-frequency sounds are less damaging than high-frequency sounds.

234.   The answer is B. *(Rosenstock, pp 23–24.)* Occupational asthma probably accounts for no more than 15 percent of cases of asthma in adults. All agents causing asthma appear to require an underlying susceptibility in the host. Occupational asthma affects mainly workers with underlying hyperreactive airways. Diagnosis is made by history and demonstration of a decline of > 10 percent in forced expiratory volume in 1 s (FEV_1) during the work shift, recovery following change in exposure, or specific inhalational challenge.

235.   The answer is D. *(Rosenstock, pp 151–157.)* Only one in five cases of occupational contact dermatitis is due to an allergic response; most are due to a direct irritation by the offending substance. Allergic contact dermatitis, however, is a lifelong problem and will almost always recur upon reexposure. Chloracne, a particularly severe form of acne, is associated with exposure to halogenated hydrocarbons. It is occasionally accompanied by hepatotoxicity or peripheral neuropathy.

236.   The answer is C. *(Rosenstock, pp 110–118.)* Exposure to cytotoxic agents, such as those used in chemotherapy, should be avoided during pregnancy. Pregnant women should avoid using *hexachlorophene*-containing soaps, which have been associated with birth defects. All personnel in intensive care units should wear lead aprons when there is portable radiography taking place, but there is no special risk associated with breast-feeding. In addition, exposure to anesthetic gases has been associated with an increased incidence of spontaneous abortions.

237.   The answer is D. *(Raffle, pp 645–653. Rosenstock, pp 33–34.)* Silicosis, usually due to inhalation of quartz dust, is a chronic, nonimmunologic lung disease characterized by the development of pulmonary nodules, which may eventually coalesce to cause progressive massive fibrosis. Eggshell calcifications in hilar lymph nodes may be seen in about 20 percent of patients. Usually, patients have been exposed to silica dusts for many years. However, an intense exposure can cause an acute and fulminant form of silicosis, which can be fatal. Occupations at risk include mining, sand-blasting (sand is largely composed of quartz), construction, and ceramics. Workers die of silicosis with a total body quartz burden of less than 1 g.

238.   The answer is C. *(Kaplan, ed 5. pp 1821–1837.)* Behavioral problems, including attention-deficit disorders and learning disabilities, are the most prevalent mental health disorders in children and occur in approximately 10 percent of children. Approximately 0.05 percent of children suffer from autism and 2 percent from mental retardation. Schizophrenia classically occurs later in life.

239.   The answer is D. *(Last, ed 12. p 851.)* Dementia is an important public health problem, especially among the institutionalized elderly. Although about half of the patients in nursing homes are demented, coronary heart disease is still the most important cause of death in this group. The diagnosis of Alzheimer's disease, which afflicts about one-half million persons in the U.S., can only be made by excluding other causes of dementia. Alzheimer's disease is more common among relatives of patients with the disease, and among persons with Down's syndrome.

240.   The answer is D. *(Kaplan, ed 5. pp 1086–1096.)* It is unknown whether the prevalence of homosexuality in the U.S. is increasing. Most observers believe that the prevalence is constant, but that increasing openness and acceptance have given the appearance of an increased prevalence. Surveys estimate that about 2 percent of women and 4 to 6 percent of men in the U.S. are homosexual.

241.   The answer is B. *(Kaplan, ed 5. pp 642–664.)* About 50 percent of the men and 70 percent of the women undergoing treatment for opiate addiction suffer from a major depressive disorder. Other common psychiatric disorders include alcoholism and antisocial personalities. Schizophrenia and mania are rare (less than 1 percent).

242.   The answer is C. *(Kaplan, ed 5. pp 1414–1427.)* Completed suicide rates are higher in white males than in white females or in nonwhites of both sexes. The suicide rate increases markedly among elderly white males but not in females or in nonwhites. Males make fewer suicide attempts than females. Suicide rates correlate not only with age, sex, and race but also with marital status (the suicide rate is higher in single, separated, divorced, or widowed persons than in those who are still married), socioeconomic status (especially among poor, elderly white males), psychiatric history, and place of residence.

243.   The answer is A. *(Wilson, ed 12. pp 2184–2185.)* Ingestion of paint chips containing lead, or soil and household dust contaminated with lead, is a substantial problem in children living in or around buildings that were erected (and painted) more than 30 or 40 years ago, when the use of lead-based paints was common. Diagnosis is easy: there are very high levels of free erythrocyte protoporphyrin (FEP), and the elevated blood level of lead confirms the diagnosis. The effects on the developing central nervous system are irreversible, but they may be the only manifestation of toxicity.

244. The answer is C. *(Kaplan, ed 5. pp 308-326.)* The President's Commission on Mental Health estimated in 1978 that 20 to 30 million Americans needed some form of help for mental and emotional disorders. Studies of patients using medical facilities indicate that 1 out of every 10 had a mental or emotional disorder.

245. The answer is A. *(Kaplan, ed 5. pp 699-705.)* Schizophrenia has a high incidence among persons in their early twenties, while affective psychosis afflicts persons in their late twenties. The annual incidence rate for schizophrenia is approximately 1 per 1,000 persons in the 15 to 24 age group. Involutional melancholia and agitated depression are specific types of depression and have their highest incidence in older persons.

246. The answer is B. *(Wilson, ed 12. p 2146.)* Significant impairment of motor coordination can occur with blood alcohol levels of only 20 to 30 mg/dL. However, the legal limit in most states is 100 mg/dL (0.1 percent). Levels of more than 300 to 400 mg/dL can be lethal. Ethanol causes more cases of toxic overdose than any other agent.

247. The answer is D. *(Kaplan, ed 5. pp 686-698.)* Most persons who have alcoholism live in the centers of large cities, and residents of cities of 50,000 or more are most likely to become alcoholics. Blacks in urban ghettos seem to be at particularly high risk. Medical students studying for board examinations are not generally considered to be at especially high risk.

248. The answer is E. *(Kaplan, ed 5. pp 686-698.)* There are 5 to 9 million alcoholics in the U.S. The incidence of alcoholism is higher among men than women; high school dropouts have the highest rate among educational subgroups. Persons with certain occupations, such as bartenders and musicians, are also at higher risk of being alcoholic. About half of the alcohol consumed in this country is drunk by 10 percent of the population.

249. The answer is E. *(Kaplan, ed 5. pp 686-698.)* Alcoholism is four times more common in families with a history of problem drinking, even if the child was adopted out of the family. About half of all alcoholics have such a family history. There is also a markedly increased risk in twins of alcoholics, especially monozygotic twins. The usual age of onset of alcoholism is between 20 and 30; it is rare for the age of onset to be after 65.

250. The answer is D. *(Kaplan, ed 5. pp 1772-1787.)* Although in several early studies, the parents of autistic children were identified frequently as professional people or as having cold or obsessive natures, or both, these findings have not been substantiated in recent studies. In fact, autistic children come from all types of backgrounds, emotional settings, and socioeconomic levels; and autism now is thought to be caused by organic biologic-neurologic factors. Three to four times as many males suffer from the disorder as females.

251.   The answer is B. *(Kaplan, ed 5. pp 1414-1427.)* The incidence of suicide increases with age, especially in whites. The highest suicide rate is found in the geriatric population. Married persons are less likely to commit suicide than single persons.

252.   The answer is C. *(Kaplan, ed 5. pp 1414-1427.)* The incidence of suicide increases with increasing age; and the rate ranges from less than 1 per 100,000 persons in the group 5 to 14 years of age to greater than 40 per 100,000 persons over 75 years of age. Suicide "attempts," however, occur mainly in young people, and the peak incidence occurs in persons who are in their late teens and early twenties. In the group 6 to 17 years of age, 25 percent of self-poisonings are said to be suicide attempts.

253.   The answer is E. *(Last, ed 12. p 1391.)* The highest risk of suicide in the U.S. is found among persons who are not religious, or who practice Buddhism. Catholics and Jews, especially if they are practicing, are at the lowest risk. Protestants are at intermediate risk.

254.   The answer is A. *(Rosenstock, p 142.)* Manganese has been associated with toxic mania. The condition is known as *locura manganica* and is characterized by emotional lability and auditory hallucinations. Lithium, of course, is used in the treatment of the mania associated with bipolar disorders.

255.   The answer is E. *(Last, ed 12. pp 953-970.)* Although there is an extensive literature on social determinants of disease, very little is known about how such factors work. Virtually all studies have found that four factors—female sex, being married, higher socioeconomic status, and a greater number of social ties—are associated with reduced mortality from nearly all diseases. These relationships are not altered by traditional risk factors (such as blood pressure), or by race or access to care.

256.   The answer is C. *(Kaplan, ed 5. pp 664-668.)* The group of people who most commonly have problems of chronic barbiturate abuse are middle-aged, middle-class persons. Heroin addicts use barbiturates as a substitute for, or an enhancer of, heroin. The most common pattern of barbiturate abuse among teen-agers is episodic use.

257.   The answer is A. *(Kaplan, ed 5. pp 2024-2034.)* Involutional depression appears during the later years of life. Hysteria most commonly occurs in adolescent and young adult women. The peak incidence for schizophrenia occurs in persons in the age group 15 to 24. Obsessive-compulsive disorder usually begins in adolescence or young adulthood.

258.   The answer is A. *(Kaplan, ed 5. pp 1096-1103.)* Only 2 percent of men who abuse their spouses are prosecuted. Although husbands who batter their wives are less educated than those who do not, educational status of women does not correlate with domestic assaults. Abuse of women in childhood is not associated with a greater probability of being assaulted by a spouse; however, women whose mothers suffered physical abuse are more likely to experience such assault.

259.   The answer is B. *(Kaplan, ed 5. pp 1854-1864.)* Anorexia nervosa is characterized by altered perception of body image leading to severe weight loss. About 95 percent of the cases occur in females. Despite the name, anorexia (loss of appetite) is rare initially. Most cases begin between ages 13 and 16.

260.   The answer is A. *(Kaplan, ed 5. pp 299-307.)* The prevalence of alcoholism and drug abuse has been shown to be five times greater among males than females. While affective disorders afflict females at a rate about twice that for males, schizophrenia occurs in males and females at about the same rate.

261.   The answer is C. *(Wilson, ed 12. p 2131.)* Panic disorders are now thought to be about as common in men as in women. They are estimated to occur in 1 to 2 percent of the population. Their usual age of onset is in the late teens or early twenties. There is a definite familial aggregation of the disorder, which is also sometimes seen in relatives of persons with affective disorders.

262.   The answer is D. *(Kaplan, ed 5. pp 852-858.)* Studies of emotional disturbances in the postpartum period have no relationship with sex of the child, parity, and a variety of other factors. Their cause is unknown, but is probably related to hormonal changes. Postpartum depression, the most common manifestation, may last up to 4 weeks. Between 20 and 40 percent of mothers report emotional or cognitive problems post partum.

263.   The answer is D. *(Kaplan, ed 5. pp 1962-1970.)* Child abuse is a major problem in the U.S.—up to a million children are maltreated each year, resulting in from 2,000 to 4,000 deaths. Child abusers come from all social classes and educational backgrounds. The mother is more commonly the abuser, perhaps because of greater contact with the child. Abusing parents are usually psychologically immature and have poor impulse control.

264.   The answer is B. *(Kaplan, ed 5. pp 642-664.)* Three to four percent of young adults (ages 18 to 25) in the U.S. have had some experience with heroin. The male to female ratio, at least in urban settings, is about 3 to 1. Use of opioids other than heroin is also more common among males. Nearly 5 percent of enlisted personnel in the military reported some use of opioids in the previous 12 months.

265. The answer is B. *(Kaplan, ed 5. pp 1810-1812.)* The cause of stuttering is not known, but genetic factors are thought to be important. Stuttering is two to three times more common in males than females and is also more common among nonwhites. The incidence is highest in young children, although there is a secondary rise in middle-age. There is a strong family tendency to stutter: up to half of the relatives of stutterers have speech dysfluency.

266. The answer is D. *(Kaplan, ed 5. pp 1414-1427.)* Attempted (unsuccessful) suicide is about 10 to 20 times more common than completed suicide. Only 1 to 2 percent of persons who attempt suicide, however, go on to commit suicide. Attempted suicide is most commonly seen in persons with hysterical or antisocial personalities.

267. The answer is D. *(Last, ed 12. pp 1371-1373.)* A similar proportion (about one in five) of men and women surveyed were affected by a significant mental disorder within the previous 6 months, but the leading diagnoses differed by sex. Phobias were the leading problem in women of all ages, affecting about 10 percent. Problems with alcohol abuse were the most common problem in men ages 18 to 64 (affecting about 10 percent). However, over the age of 65, cognitive impairment was the leading problem: it affected almost 6 percent of men, whereas only 3 percent of men over 65 admitted problems with alcohol. The majority of persons whose responses indicated one or more mental health disorders were not receiving any mental health care.

268. The answer is D. *(Rosenstock, pp 88-89.)* Occupational exposures, especially to aniline dyes and related organic nitrogen compounds, are thought to be responsible for about 20 percent of all cases of bladder cancer (smoking is the other major risk factor). There is usually a long latent period, from 15 to 40 years, between exposure and disease. Workers in the rubber industry are exposed to β-naphthylamine, an antioxidant and known bladder carcinogen; some physicians recommend that such workers undergo cytologic examination of their urine on a regular basis.

269. The answer is C. *(Green, ed 6. pp 328-329.)* Approximately 50 percent of motor vehicle fatalities are associated with at least one driver's having a blood alcohol level over 0.1 percent, a level that makes one legally intoxicated. The probability of an automobile crash increases significantly with increasing blood levels of alcohol. Other important variables associated with motor vehicle injuries include age and sex of the driver and vehicle size. Males 15 to 24 years of age have high fatality-to-injury ratios, as do older people who are less able to survive injuries.

Drivers of smaller cars are less protected from injuries than are drivers of larger cars. Airbags are advocated as a means to passively protect all drivers.

270-273.   The answers are: 270-B, 271-C, 272-A, 273-D. *(Benenson, ed 15. pp 115-117, 182-185, 197-200, 247-250. Last, ed 12. p 123.)* Hepatitis A virus spreads readily in day-care centers, particularly those caring for toddlers in diapers. It usually causes mild or no disease in the children, but may cause significant morbidity in adult contacts.

Cytomegalovirus (CMV) is very common in children in day-care centers; in one study more than half of the children excreted CMV over the course of a year, compared with less than 10 percent of children cared for at home. Most infections are asymptomatic, but infection of the fetus can cause microcephaly, mental retardation, deafness, and death.

Giardiasis affects both children and their adult contacts. Symptoms may be absent, mild, or severe and may include diarrhea, bloating, fat malabsorption, and weight loss. Diagnosis is by identification of cysts or trophozoites in the stool (but false negatives are frequent), or by finding trophozoites in duodenal fluid, either by direct aspiration or with a string test.

Leptospirosis is a systemic illness caused by the spirochete *Leptospira interrogans* and is acquired by contact of abraded skin or mucous membranes with fresh water contaminated with the urine of infected animals. Transmission from person to person is rare. Doxycycline is effective treatment when given early in the course.

274-276.   The answers are: 274-D, 275-B, 276-C. *(Mausner, ed 2. pp 78-79, 85-87.)* Meningococcal meningitis, because of its severity and the fear of epidemics, is reportable in all states. Reporting of meningococcal meningitis to local and state health departments by physicians tends to be more complete than reporting of less severe diseases such as measles, German measles, or salmonellosis. Many states improve the completeness of their infectious disease surveillance by requiring all diagnostic laboratories to report the isolation of certain pathogenic microbes.

The incidence and prevalence of chronic diseases such as arthritis are difficult to determine because patients who have arthritis often do not need hospitalization. The National Health Interview Survey uses data obtained by conducting household surveys of defined populations and attempts continuously to provide data on the health status and needs of the country.

In several states and foreign countries, all newly diagnosed cases of cancer that occur in a defined geographic area are reported to a cancer registry and then followed by the registry until death of the patients. Such registries provide very important information on the incidence, prevalence, and survival rates of different types of cancers. In addition, the registries provide a source of cases for case-control studies and other research.

277–280.   The answers are: 277–B, 278–D, 279–A, 280–C. *(Benenson, ed 15. pp 66, 83, 224, 271, 330, 347–348, 353–354, 381–382, 386, 392, 411–417, 486.)* Rabies, psittacosis, and salmonellosis are zoonoses, that is, infections transmitted from animals to humans. The reservoirs of rabies include domestic and wild canines, cats, skunks, raccoons, bats, and other biting mammals. Psittacosis is a zoonosis involving birds such as parakeets, parrots, pigeons, turkeys, and other domestic fowl. *Salmonella* species infect poultry, rodents, dogs, cats, and birds (*S. typhi* is an exception in that no animal hosts are known).

Influenza, yellow fever, and chickenpox are caused by viruses. The diseases differ significantly in their clinical manifestations: influenza is an acute respiratory tract infection; chickenpox is characterized by fever and a typical skin rash; and yellow fever is a severe disseminated viral infection with jaundice.

Pneumococcus, Streptococcus, and *Brucella* are genera of bacteria. Microbes of the first two genera are pathogens responsible for respiratory tract infections in humans. *Brucella* is a cause of widespread zoonoses in cattle, pigs, goats, and sheep, but only occasionally causes human disease.

Measles, shigellosis, and scabies can be transmitted directly from person to person. Measles virus is spread in the respiratory secretions of infected persons; shigellosis is easily caused by ingestion of only a few hundred *Shigella* bacteria and can be spread from person to person by the fecal-oral route; and scabies, a skin infection caused by the mite *Sarcoptes scabiei*, is spread by direct person-to-person contact, often during sexual activity.

281–284.   The answers are: 281–A, 282–B, 283–D, 284–C. *(Mausner, ed 2. pp 268–269.)* *Immunogenicity* is a term that describes the ability of a microbe or purified antigen to induce specific antibody production in a host as a result of infection or immunization. For example, measles virus is very immunogenic because most persons develop neutralizing antibody, which persists for life following a single infection.

Pathogenicity is the capacity of a microbe to cause symptomatic illness in an infected host. The enormous numbers of nonpathogenic bacteria (up to 10^{10} per gram of colonic contents) present in the human body and the normal flora on the human body's external surfaces do not cause disease.

Virulence refers to the severity of illness produced by a microbe and is measured by the percentage of severe or fatal cases. Virulence may vary depending on the defenses of the host; for example, malnutrition impairs defenses against infection. In malnourished children, measles has a case-fatality rate of up to 10 percent compared with less than 0.1 percent in well-nourished children.

Contagiousness of a microbe refers to the ability of a microbe to spread in a population of exposed susceptible persons. The secondary attack rate, that is, the incidence of a disease in contacts of a case, often is used to assess contagiousness.

285-288.   The answers are: 285-A, 286-C, 287-B, 288-D. *(Benenson, ed 15. pp 61-66, 130-132, 170-175.)* Staphylococcal food poisoning is caused by a heat-stable enterotoxin produced when staphylococci multiply in food. The incubation period is usually 2 to 4 h, and the illness is characterized by the sudden onset of severe nausea, vomiting, cramps, prostration, and diarrhea.

Botulism is caused by a toxin produced by *Clostridium botulinum.* The toxin, produced anaerobically in improperly processed foods, is neurotoxic, and the illness is characterized by progressive descending muscle paralysis. Botulism may lead to death from respiratory failure.

Food poisoning caused by *Clostridium perfringens* usually has an incubation period of 10 to 12 h and is characterized by abrupt onset of abdominal colic followed by diarrhea. Vomiting is unusual, and the disease is usually of short duration. Outbreaks result from contamination of food during preparation and by improper cooking and storage; these circumstances allow bacteria to multiply.

Most cases of traveler's diarrhea are caused by enterotoxin-producing strains of *Escherichia coli.* Although the mechanism of action of *E. coli* enterotoxin is similar to that of cholera enterotoxin, disease due to the former is usually not as severe. Disease due to *E. coli* enterotoxin is most common in regions of the world where adequate sanitation and pure water supplies are absent.

289-292.   The answers are: 289-A, 290-E, 291-C, 292-B. *(Wilson, ed 12. pp 1437, 1463-1464, 1475, 1834-1835.)* Gout is caused by the deposition of urate crystals in a joint. It is almost always associated with hyperuricemia, which is frequently caused by diuretic therapy used in the treatment of hypertension or congestive heart failure. It can also be idiopathic (caused by either overproduction or underexcretion of uric acid), or associated with underlying malignancy or renal disease.

Although rheumatoid arthritis is the most common and severe form of arthritis in children, its *usual* onset is between 35 and 50 years of age. Rheumatoid arthritis is more common in women than men, and among relatives of patients with the disease. The cause of this potentially devastating disease is unknown. Certain types of juvenile rheumatoid arthritis are associated with HLA-B27. Other arthritides associated with HLA-B27 include ankylosing spondylitis, reactive arthritis, and Reiter's syndrome.

Osteoarthritis afflicts the majority of all persons over the age of 75 years and is by far the most common form of arthritis in all regions of the U.S.

Although sarcoid may be slightly more common in the southeastern U.S. than in other regions of the country, it is still a rare disease. In addition, only about one-quarter to one-half of all patients with sarcoid have arthritis.

293-296.   The answers are: 293-C, 294-B, 295-C, 296-B. *(Wilson, ed 12. pp 692, 1351, 1457.)* The hepatitis B virus, a mostly double-stranded DNA virus, has been associated with both hepatomas and polyarteritis nodosa. Hepatomas are most commonly seen among persons who have been lifelong carriers of hepatitis B surface antigen (HBsAg), usually because they were infected in infancy or early childhood. There may be associated integration of the HBV genome into hepatocytes. Polyarteritis nodosa (PAN) is a systemic vasculitis of small- and medium-sized arteries, classically manifested by fever, abdominal pain, and hematuria. The nature of the relationship between the hepatitis B virus and PAN is not clear; however, approximately 30 percent of patients with PAN are HBsAg positive.

Epstein-Barr virus, a double-stranded DNA virus in the herpes family, is the cause of infectious mononucleosis. High titers of antibody to certain of the viral antigens are seen in the vast majority of patients with anaplastic nasopharyngeal cancer (a relatively common cancer in southeast China), and with Burkitt lymphoma in Africa and New Guinea. Interestingly, there does not seem to be a relationship between Burkitt lymphoma and EBV in the United States.

Hepatitis A virus, adenovirus, and cytomegalovirus are not associated with any particular chronic diseases, though CMV infections are more common among persons who are immunosuppressed.

297–301. The answers are: 297-B, 298-A, 299-E, 300-D, 301-C. *(Last, ed 12. pp 562–569. Wilson, ed 12. pp 1056–1063.)* Occupational exposure to beryllium dust is a hazard to workers in the manufacturing environments of aircraft assembly, metallurgical processes, and ceramics. Focal, noncaseating granulomas are the consequence of long exposure to beryllium dust. These are followed by a diffuse interstitial fibrosis that reduces lung volume, decreases gas transport, and causes dyspnea and nonproductive cough.

Bagassosis is due to inhalation of spores of microorganisms, especially *Thermoactinomyces*. It is mainly seen in workers in the sugar cane processing industry.

The acute symptoms of byssinosis occur in many workers after years of breathing air containing dusts of cotton, flax, or hemp and consist of chest tightness, cough, and wheezing. In persons who have chronic byssinosis, the pulmonary damage is irreversible. Airways are severely obstructed and lack normal elastic recoil.

Rheumatoid pneumoconiosis, or Caplan's syndrome, is seen in coal workers. Progressive massive fibrosis, consisting of a network of reticular fibers and coal dust deposits, is accompanied by seropositive rheumatoid arthritis. (Although first described with coal workers' pneumoconiosis, seropositive rheumatoid arthritis has now been described with other occupational lung diseases.)

Siderosis is caused by chronic inhalation of iron oxide dust that is airborne in the work environments of welders. Pulmonary tissue responses are not significant, but serious impairment of pulmonary function may result from fibrosis, the extent of which is determined by the silica content of the inhaled iron dust.

The most common chronic pulmonary disease related to inorganic dust is asbestosis, which affects not only the worker but also the family (e.g., when the worker shakes work clothes) and the neighborhood.

302-306. The answers are: 302-A, 303-E, 304-D, 305-B, 306-C. *(Wilson, ed 12. pp 625-626, 635, 745, 749, 1326-1327.)* Although most occupational diseases are not infectious in origin, it is important to be aware of those that are. Butchers, meat packers, farmers, and livestock handlers are at risk of developing brucellosis, a febrile illness caused by several species of *Brucella*, a gram-negative coccobacillus. Occupational infection usually results from inoculation through abraded skin or mucous membranes; gloves and goggles can prevent this form of spread. Infection may also result from ingestion of raw milk or animal tissues. Treatment is with tetracycline.

Sporotrichosis is caused by the fungus *Sporothrix schenckii*, a common plant saprophyte. Infection is usually caused by inoculation of the organism into a wound, such as that caused by a rose thorn. It usually causes a lymphangitic disease, with a localized papule and distant nodules. Treatment is with oral potassium iodide.

Air-conditioning workers and others (such as hospital patients) exposed to air from cooling ducts containing water are susceptible to legionellosis, a severe pneumonia caused by *Legionella pneumophila*. *L. pneumophila* is a gram-negative rod that inhabits warm, moist areas, such as cooling systems. It is named after a famous epidemic that occurred in 1976 at an American Legion convention in Philadelphia, in which at least 220 people were infected with a (then) mysterious illness. Treatment is with erythromycin.

Dentists and other health workers exposed to blood and other body fluids are at risk for hepatitis B, a viral infection. The incubation period is 1 to 4 months. There is no treatment, but the disease can be prevented by immunization.

Spelunkers are at risk for histoplasmosis, a fungal infection caused by *Histoplasma capsulatum*. *H. capsulatum* grows in soil, particularly that enriched by bird or bat excrement (the reason it is found in caves). Infection, which is more common in the central and southeastern U.S., is usually asymptomatic but may cause a chronic pulmonary disease that mimics tuberculosis. Treatment is with ketoconazole or amphotericin B.

307-311. The answers are: 307-C, 308-A, 309-A, 310-D, 311-B. *(Rosenstock, pp 174, 230, 247, 253.)* Some of the new media used by artists today are hazardous materials that include solvents and paints composed of vinyl acrylic acid, vinyl chloride, vinyl acetate, ethyl silicate, and pyroxylin. Contact with and inhalation of such substances may cause dermatitis and systemic toxic reactions, respectively. These materials are especially hazardous if they burn; extremely toxic gases, including hydrogen cyanide, may be released.

The principal health hazard associated with pottery manufacture is due to inhalation of silica dust generated during crushing and screening operations. Workers in glass manufacturing plants constitute another occupational group chronically exposed to silica dust. The use of wet sand in the manufacturing process reduces the hazard of developing silicosis, but the hazard is still present.

Workers in many different types of unventilated settings, such as sewers and oil tanks, are exposed to hydrogen sulfide. This gas, which smells like rotten eggs, can cause blockade of cellular respiration in high doses.

In the production of molds and castings in foundries, the occupational environment is characterized by conditions of excessive noise, vibration, and heat, as well as the presence of air contaminants.

312–315.   The answers are: 312-E, 313-E, 314-B, 315-A. *(Last, ed 12. pp 1125–1132.)* Deaths associated with automobile crashes account for about 20 percent of all deaths in children 1 to 14 years old. In this age group, injuries of all types caused almost 50 percent of all deaths. Cancer is the second leading cause of death. One-third of the deaths in the age group 14 to 24 are due to automobile crashes. Cancer is also the second leading cause of death in this age group. The leading cause of death in the group 25 to 44 years of age is cancer, only slightly ahead of heart disease. Heart disease is the leading cause of death for adults in the group 45 to 64 years of age. For these adults, cancer is the second leading cause of death and the death rate for stroke exceeds that for automobile crashes. The only infectious disease listed among the ten leading causes of death is pneumonia, which outranks automobile crashes as a cause of death only in infants less than 1 year of age and in adults over 65 years of age.

316–320.   The answers are: 316-C, 317-E, 318-D, 319-D, 320-B. *(Last, ed 12. pp 587–615, 617–702.)* Of the 70,000 chemicals currently in commercial production, only 1,400 (2 percent) have been tested for their carcinogenicity. Of these, about 30 have been found by direct observations of exposed human populations to cause cancer. *β-Naphthylamine*, an aromatic amine used to produce dyes, rodenticides, and many other chemicals, has been identified as an agent that causes bladder cancer. *Benzene*, or benzole, is used in the production of coal tar derivatives, solvents, paints, and printing inks, and as a cleaning agent by auto mechanics. Based on epidemiologic evidence, benzene is regarded as a causative agent of leukemia and lymphoma. Vapors of *nickel*, a component of many alloys, and nickel sulfides, when inhaled over long periods of time, have been cited as a cause of cancer of the nasal cavities and the lungs. The carcinogenicity of nickel is based partly on studies of nickel refinery workers, in whom these cancers developed more than 20 years after exposure. Also, workers in the *chromate*-producing industries are at high risk of developing cancer of the nasal cavities and lungs. *Vinyl chloride*, a gas at room temperature, has been shown to cause cancer of the liver, brain, and lungs. Skin cancer is induced by occupational exposure to arsenic compounds, soot, tars, and oils, as well as by ultraviolet light.

321–324.   The answers are: 321-D, 322-C, 323-B, 324-C. *(Last, ed 12. pp 587–615, 617–702.)* Coal workers' pneumoconiosis (black lung disease) is chronic fibrosis of the lung caused by inhalation of coal dust. The disease can be prevented by reducing levels of coal dust in mines. The United States Coal Mine Health and Safety Act of 1969 and the "Black Lung Law" of 1972 provide compensation for victims of the disease and their dependents.

Methyl mercury concentrates in red blood cells and in nerve cells and can lead to severe and fatal neurologic disease. Symptoms include paresthesia, ataxia, visual disturbances, deafness, personality changes, and spasticity. The largest known incident of methyl mercury poisoning occurred in the regions near Minamata Bay in Japan. Almost 4,000 cases have been identified, all resulting from pollution of the bay by effluent from local chemical plants and consequent contamination of the bay's fish.

Sulfur dioxide by itself may not cause chronic bronchitis and emphysema. However, exposure to sulfur dioxide, in combination with suspended particulates and active chemicals in smog, has been associated with increased symptoms of chronic bronchitis.

Occupational exposure to thallium is associated with a characteristic triad: gastroenteritis, polyneuropathy, and hair loss. The neuropathy may persist. Most cases are associated with the use or manufacture of thallium-containing rodenticides, although thallium is used in several industrial and mining processes.

325-328.   The answers are: 325-C, 326-A, 327-A, 328-C. *(Last, ed 12. pp 1151-1155. Wilson, ed 12. pp 1233, 1248, 1922, 2160.)* Alcohol and tobacco both cause esophageal cancer. The risk of the disease is increased in smokers about fivefold and in drinkers about tenfold. Persons who both smoke and drink are also at increased risk of oral cancers.

Carcinogens contained in tobacco smoke have been found in cervical mucus, perhaps explaining the increased risk of cervical cancer in smokers. Cigarette smoking increases the incidence of duodenal ulcers and slows their healing. Studies have shown that failure to quit smoking may prevent ulcer healing even in patients who are otherwise appropriately treated. Alcohol is associated with gastritis and gastric ulcer disease, but not with duodenal ulcer disease.

Osteoporotic hip fractures are more prevalent in thin women who smoke and in alcoholics. The biologic explanation for these epidemiologic findings is uncertain. Other important risk factors include advanced age, female sex, and white race.

Primary and Secondary Prevention of Specific Illnesses

DIRECTIONS: Each question below contains five suggested responses. Select the **one best** response to each question.

329. Correct statements concerning fluoridation of drinking water include all the following EXCEPT

(A) fluoridation of drinking water reduces caries by about 50 percent
(B) the advisability of fluoridation is still controversial among dental public health experts
(C) the optimum concentration of fluoride in public drinking water depends on the average daily air temperature of the community served
(D) fluorosis, a white or brown discoloration of the teeth from too much fluoride, often occurs if the concentration of fluoride exceeds 2 to 3 parts per million (ppm)
(E) most people cannot taste fluoride at concentrations of 1 ppm

330. True statements regarding type B *Haemophilus influenzae* include all the following EXCEPT

(A) it is a more important cause of mortality in children than in adults
(B) polysaccharide vaccine conjugated with diphtheria toxoid should be given to children beginning at 2 months of age
(C) it is the most common cause of acute otitis media in children
(D) it is the major cause of acute epiglottitis
(E) it is resistant to ampicillin in over 15 percent of cases

DBEBBC

118

331. Which of the following prenatal screening tests is recommended for all pregnant women?

(A) Hemoglobin electrophoresis
(B) Hepatitis B surface antigen
(C) HIV antibody
(D) Ultrasound
(E) None of the above

332. Which of the following statements concerning the ELISA test for the presence of antibodies to the human immunodeficiency virus (HIV; the AIDS virus) is true?

(A) Only about 10 percent of those with antibodies to the virus (i.e., a true positive ELISA test) will get AIDS
(B) The presence of antibody correlates well with protective immunity
(C) The ELISA test has a low positive predictive value when low-risk populations are screened
(D) False positive tests sometimes occur in patients with far-advanced AIDS
(E) People whose ELISA test is negative cannot transmit HIV to others

333. Correct statements concerning iron requirements include all the following EXCEPT

(A) iron requirements are satisfied by cow's milk
(B) iron requirements of women decrease after menopause
(C) iron requirements are the same in adult men and postmenopausal women
(D) iron requirements increase during pregnancy
(E) patients with thalassemia do not need extra iron

334. Clinical trials of the management of patients with coronary heart disease have shown that all the following are true EXCEPT

(A) treatment with calcium channel blockers reduces mortality
(B) treatment with beta blockers reduces mortality
(C) treatment with aspirin reduces mortality
(D) coronary artery bypass grafting prolongs life in patients with three-vessel coronary artery disease and poor left ventricular function
(E) nitrates are useful in symptomatic relief of angina

335. All the following statements regarding the trace element iodine are true EXCEPT

(A) adequate intake of iodine is essential because it is a component of several enzymes involved in intermediary metabolism
(B) deficiency develops primarily in areas where the level of iodine in the soil is insufficient
(C) it is extremely toxic at high doses
(D) deficiency leads to goiter, but rarely to hypothyroidism
(E) iodine supplements are recommended for persons who may be exposed to radioactive fallout

336. Correct statements regarding hepatitis B include all the following EXCEPT

(A) vertical transmission is a major public health problem in Asia
(B) vertical transmission can be prevented by hepatitis B immune globulin and hepatitis B vaccine
(C) persons working in dialysis units are at particularly high risk of occupational exposure
(D) transmission is primarily via the fecal-oral route in the United States
(E) chronic carriers are at increased risk of hepatocellular carcinoma

337. Hospital employees involved in patient care are at increased risk both of acquiring and of transmitting certain infections. Vaccines recommended for such workers include

(A) BCG vaccine
(B) typhoid vaccine
(C) pneumococcal polysaccharide vaccine
(D) rubella vaccine
(E) none of the above

338. Which of the following statements about the risks and benefits of postmenopausal hormonal replacement therapy is true?

(A) The increased risk of endometrial cancer is especially high among women using combination preparations (estrogen and progestin)
(B) The main potential benefit is a reduced risk of hip fracture
(C) Most studies have shown a reduced risk of breast cancer among women using estrogen-only preparations
(D) Most studies have shown a beneficial effect on mortality from coronary heart disease
(E) There is a slightly increased risk of pulmonary embolism

339. The case-fatality rate of cholera is currently less than 1 percent. Major factors responsible for this low case-fatality rate include

(A) treatment with tetracycline or other antibiotics
(B) mass immunization in endemic regions
(C) widespread use of intravenous hydration
(D) chlorination of water supplies in endemic regions
(E) none of the above

340. Immunization of preschool children with diphtheria toxoid results in

(A) protection against the diphtheria carrier state
(B) lifelong immunity against diphtheria
(C) detectable antitoxin for about 10 years
(D) frequent adverse reactions
(E) protection against infection of the respiratory tract by *Corynebacterium diphtheriae*

341. Epidemics of typhus fever have been associated with war and famine for several centuries. What factor was most important in the control of such epidemics following the end of World War II?

(A) Eradication of *Anopheles* mosquitoes
(B) Improved sanitation practices
(C) Improved methods for handling food supplies
(D) Disinfestation by use of DDT
(E) Mass therapy with antibiotics

342. The administration of a single injection of live attenuated measles vaccine results in

(A) seroconversion in 95 percent of susceptible children
(B) the induction of active immunity that lasts less than 5 years
(C) postimmunization encephalitis in 0.1 percent of recipients
(D) subacute sclerosing panencephalitis in 0.017 percent of recipients
(E) no significant risk to children with leukemia

343. Preventive treatment with isoniazid (isonicotinic acid hydrazide) is recommended for all the following groups EXCEPT

(A) young adults in whom a positive tuberculin test is demonstrated
(B) children under age 3 in whom a positive tuberculin test is demonstrated
(C) all members of a household in which one member has an active case of tuberculosis
(D) children with atypical mycobacterial infection
(E) nursing mothers with positive tuberculin skin tests

344. Passive immunization is the major means of prevention of which of the following diseases?

(A) Influenza
(B) German measles
(C) Mumps
(D) Viral hepatitis type A
(E) None of the above

545. Reasons to treat gonorrhea with oral tetracycline 500 mg qid for 7 days—rather than with oral ampicillin 3.5 g plus oral probenecid 1 g taken at one time—include

(A) lower frequency of side effects
(B) better coverage of *Chlamydia trachomatis*
(C) greater safety in case of pregnancy
(D) enhanced compliance
(E) none of the above

346. Which of the following statements concerning skin testing for tuberculosis is correct?

(A) All children should be tested yearly with intermediate-strength purified protein derivative (PPD)
(B) Children with positive tests do not require treatment if their chest x-ray is negative
(C) Compared with children, adults with tuberculosis are much less likely to be contagious
(D) Atypical mycobacteria may cause false positive results
(E) None of the above

347. Adverse reactions reported following administration of pertussis vaccine include

(A) arthus reaction
(B) seizures
(C) hyperglycemia
(D) hypothermia
(E) none of the above

348. Correct statements about hepatitis B virus include all the following EXCEPT

(A) the incubation period for hepatitis B is longer than that for hepatitis A
(B) prevention of hepatitis B infection can be accomplished by means of hyperimmune globulin or vaccine
(C) specific diagnostic tests are not available for hepatitis B
(D) hepatitis B virus may persist in the blood for years
(E) the recombinant vaccine uses hepatitis B surface antigen

349. Prevention of human brucellosis depends on

(A) pasteurization of dairy products derived from goats, sheep, or cows
(B) treatment of human cases
(C) control of the insect vector
(D) immunization of farmers and slaughterhouse workers
(E) none of the above

350. Influenza vaccine is generally recommended for which of the following groups?

(A) All persons over 55 years of age
(B) School-age children
(C) All persons with severe pulmonary disorders regardless of age
(D) Pregnant women
(E) None of the above

351. Often, visual disturbances and sore throat are the first symptoms in cases of botulism. Other characteristics of this form of intoxication are described by all the following statements EXCEPT

(A) in the United States, most cases result from inadequate processing of home-canned foods
(B) the incubation period is usually 12 to 36 h
(C) toxins produced by *Clostridium botulinum* are destroyed by boiling
(D) death is most often the result of the effect of the toxin on the myocardium
(E) it should be treated with antitoxin

352. Which of the following statements regarding herpes simplex virus, type 2 (HSV-2), is correct?

(A) Infections with HSV-2 are almost always symptomatic
(B) Transmission from mother to infant is generally transplacental
(C) HSV infection is an early sign of the acquired immunodeficiency syndrome
(D) Neonates with cutaneous disease should receive antiviral therapy regardless of whether there is evidence of dissemination
(E) None of the above

353. All the following statements about diphtheria, pertussis, and tetanus are true EXCEPT

(A) immunization against the three diseases should be started at 2 months of age
(B) most adults are not immune to pertussis
(C) the pertussis vaccine is a toxoid that is relatively frequently associated with adverse effects
(D) tetanus immune globulin should be given for dirty wounds only if the patient's tetanus immunizations are not up to date
(E) adults should receive a diphtheria booster at the time of their tetanus boosters (as a Td)

354. Effective means of preventing trichinosis in humans include

(A) cooking pork and pork products to ensure that all parts of the meat reach a temperature of at least 40°C (104° F)
(B) attention to proper disposal of hog feces
(C) prohibiting the marketing of garbage-fed hogs
(D) skin testing of hogs with *Trichinella* antigen prior to slaughter
(E) none of the above

355. True statements about Lyme disease include

(A) it is caused by an arthropod-borne virus (arbovirus)
(B) it is associated with a characteristic skin rash, called erythema marginatum centrificum (EMC)
(C) it occurs primarily in the Rocky Mountain states of the U.S.
(D) it may involve the heart and the central nervous system, as well as joints
(E) none of the above

356. Diseases that are transmitted chiefly from person to person include

(A) California encephalitis
(B) St. Louis encephalitis
(C) lymphocytic choriomeningitis
(D) meningococcal meningitis
(E) none of the above

357. In the United States, exfoliative cytology is the most commonly used test for detection of cancer of the

(A) skin
(B) breast
(C) stomach
(D) colon
(E) cervix

358. Major risk factors for coronary artery disease include all the following EXCEPT

(A) an elevated low-density lipoprotein (LDL) level
(B) an elevated high-density lipoprotein (HDL) level
(C) hypertension
(D) cigarette smoking
(E) male sex

359. Which of the following statements about the treatment of hypertension is true?

(A) Treating hypertension has been shown to reduce the incidence of stroke
(B) Treating mild-to-moderate hypertension has been shown to reduce the incidence of coronary heart disease
(C) Most persons with hypertension in the U.S. are not aware that they have high blood pressure
(D) No study has ever demonstrated a benefit from treating hypertension in men
(E) No study has ever demonstrated a benefit from treating hypertension in women

360. All the following techniques are considered useful in screening for cancer in asymptomatic persons EXCEPT

(A) breast self-examination in a 45-year-old woman
(B) mammography in a 45-year-old woman
(C) mammography in a 55-year-old woman
(D) Pap smear in a 55-year-old female smoker
(E) chest radiography in a 55-year-old male smoker

361. A 40-year-old man with a total cholesterol of 300 mg/dL, a triglyceride of 200 mg/dL, and an HDL cholesterol of 40 mg/dL (after an overnight fast) has an LDL cholesterol of approximately

(A) 260 mg/dL
(B) 220 mg/dL
(C) 160 mg/dL
(D) 140 mg/dL
(E) 60 mg/dL

362. All the following are dietary determinants of plasma lipid levels EXCEPT

(A) alcohol
(B) total calories
(C) cholesterol
(D) saturated fat
(E) vitamin E

363. Use of postmenopausal estrogens has been consistently associated with

(A) an increased risk of endometrial cancer
(B) a decreased risk of breast cancer
(C) an increased risk of osteoporotic fractures
(D) an increased risk of coronary heart disease
(E) an increased incidence of liver cancer

364. Which of the following statements about blood pressure is true?

(A) Isolated systolic hypertension is defined as a systolic blood pressure above 200 mmHg with a normal diastolic blood pressure
(B) Isolated systolic hypertension is a risk factor for stroke
(C) Diastolic blood pressure is a more important predictor of incidence of coronary heart disease than is systolic blood pressure
(D) The prevalence of isolated systolic hypertension increases with age in men but not in women
(E) The prevalence of isolated systolic hypertension peaks between ages 60 and 70

365. Which of the following statements about inflammatory bowel disease is true?

(A) The incidence of ulcerative colitis is lower in Jews
(B) Total colectomy to prevent malignancy is recommended for all persons who have had ulcerative colitis for more than 20 years
(C) The incidence of Crohn's disease is increased in Jews
(D) Total colectomy to prevent malignancy is recommended for all persons who have had Crohn's disease of the colon for more than 20 years
(E) Both Crohn's disease and ulcerative colitis are more common in men than in women

366. The prognosis for patients with coronary artery disease is related to all the following EXCEPT

(A) serum cholesterol level
(B) left ventricular function
(C) family history of heart disease
(D) degree of coronary artery stenosis
(E) severity of ischemia

367. The major environmental source of lead absorbed in the human bloodstream is

(A) air
(B) water
(C) lead-based paint
(D) food
(E) none of the above

368. All the following statements about occupational health in the U.S. are true EXCEPT

(A) there are over 20,000 toxic substances in use
(B) occupational diseases are responsible for about 100,000 deaths annually
(C) there are about 400,000 new cases of occupational disease annually
(D) occupational exposures are responsible for about half of all deaths caused by chronic obstructive pulmonary disease
(E) occupational exposures are responsible for about 5 to 10 percent of all cancer deaths

369. The key factors involved in the prevention of back injuries include all the following EXCEPT

(A) the prevention of the first injury, since subsequent injuries are more likely to occur
(B) the adjustment of an uncomfortable load once it has been lifted
(C) the development of weight-lifting limits adjusted for the age and physical condition of workers
(D) the requirement of preemployment radiographs of the lumbosacral spine
(E) mechanical lifting devices

370. The threshold limit value (TLV) is used by industries and government agencies to describe the allowable amount of a toxic chemical to which persons may be occupationally exposed. This standard is correctly described by which of the following statements?

(A) It has been established for most chemicals in use by industry
(B) It is based on average exposure, so that workers can be exposed to levels above the established TLV at times during the work day
(C) It takes into account the interaction of a number of toxic chemicals present simultaneously in the same environment
(D) It does not require a monitoring system to evaluate the levels of the chemical in the worker's environment
(E) None of the above

371. Depression can be caused or exacerbated by drugs used in the treatment of hypertension. Which of the following statements about this type of depression is true?

(A) Nearly all patients being treated with alpha methyldopa report depression
(B) Drug-related depression is often permanent, even if the drug is discontinued
(C) Most patients with drug-induced depression have an underlying psychologic cause of depression as well
(D) The prevalance of depression is related to the degree of lowering of blood pressure
(E) None of the above

372. Infants born to mothers who are heavy drinkers are at increased risk of which of the following problems?

(A) Mental retardation
(B) Chronic liver disease
(C) Excessive birth weight
(D) Chorioretinitis
(E) Deafness

373. Characteristic signs or symptoms of kwashiorkor include all the following EXCEPT

(A) hypoalbuminemia
(B) loss of subcutaneous fat
(C) edema
(D) diarrhea
(E) ulcerated skin lesions

374. Which of the following statements about the use of nicotine-containing chewing gum to help cigarette smokers quit smoking is true?

(A) It is most successful in persons who are not addicted to nicotine
(B) It is most successful in persons with low levels of addiction to nicotine
(C) It is most successful in persons with moderate levels of addiction to nicotine
(D) It is most successful in persons with high levels of addiction to nicotine
(E) Its success is unrelated to the degree of nicotine addiction

375. Causative factors for organic brain syndrome that have been virtually eliminated as a result of the practice of preventive medicine include

(A) syphilis
(B) lead
(C) vitamin C deficiency
(D) hallucinogenic drugs
(E) none of the above

DIRECTIONS: Each group of questions below consists of lettered headings followed by a set of numbered items. For each numbered item select the **one** lettered heading with which it is **most** closely associated. Each lettered heading may be used **once, more than once, or not at all.**

Questions 376–379

Match each set of symptoms and signs with the dietary deficiency.

(A) Vitamin A deficiency
(B) Thiamine deficiency
(C) Vitamin C deficiency
(D) Vitamin D deficiency
(E) Niacin deficiency

376. Petechiae, sore gums, hematuria, and bone or joint pain

377. Dermatitis, diarrhea, and delirium

378. Edema, neuropathy, and myocardial failure

379. Conjunctival xerosis, hyperkeratosis, and keratomalacia

Questions 380–384

For each preventive health measure or concern, select the age range with which it is associated.

(A) Birth to 18 months
(B) Ages 2 to 6
(C) Ages 7 to 12
(D) Ages 13 to 18

380. Initial blood pressure screening

381. Initial dental visit

382. Tetanus-diphtheria (Td) booster

383. Routine blood testing

384. Suicide as a leading cause of death

Questions 385–388

Match each of the descriptions below with the correct worm.

(A) *Necator americanus* (hookworm)
(B) *Ascaris lumbricoides* (roundworm)
(C) *Strongyloides stercoralis*
(D) *Taenia solium* (pork tapeworm)
(E) *Trichuris trichiura* (whipworm)

385. Infection follows ingestion of embryonated eggs, which mature into larvae in the intestine, then migrate to the lungs to mature further

386. Infection of man by this worm in the larval stage is termed *cysticercosis*

387. Intestinal autoinfection may lead to increasing worm burden and dissemination

388. Acquired when infective larvae penetrate the skin; main symptoms are due to iron deficiency

Questions 389–392

For each description below, match the appropriate arthropod parasite.

(A) *Sarcoptes scabiei*
(B) *Pediculus humanus capitis*
(C) *Pediculus humanus corporis*
(D) *Phthirius pubis*
(E) None of the above

389. Vector for epidemic typhus and relapsing fever

390. Epidemics in school children; best treated with a 1% permethrin preparation

391. Vector for Lyme disease

392. Burrows under the skin

Questions 393–396

Match each description to the proper trace element.

(A) Chromium
(B) Cobalt
(C) Copper
(D) Selenium
(E) Zinc

393. Works closely with vitamin E as an antioxidant

394. Cofactor for many enzymes; essential for normal sense of taste

395. Cofactor for vitamin B_{12}

396. Works with insulin allowing uptake of glucose; deficiency may lead to diabetes

Questions 397–401

Match the following ethnic groups with the disease for which it would be most appropriate to institute a screening program.

(A) Alpha thalassemia
(B) Beta thalassemia
(C) Cystic fibrosis
(D) Hemophilia
(E) Tay-Sachs disease

397. Italians

398. Chinese

399. Ashkenazic Jews

400. Greeks

401. Germans

Questions 402–405

For each situation below, choose the approximate risk of transmission of the human immunodeficiency virus (HIV).

(A) 1/2 or more
(B) 1/10
(C) 1/500
(D) 1/10,000
(E) 1/100,000 or less

402. Risk to a woman of a single episode of penile-vaginal intercourse with an infected (HIV-positive) man not using a condom

403. Risk to a woman of 10 episodes of penile-vaginal intercourse with a man who does not belong to any high-risk group and whose HIV serostatus is unknown

404. Risk to a hospital worker following a single needle-stick from an HIV-infected patient

405. Risk to a recipient of a unit of blood from an HIV-positive donor

Questions 406–409

For each disease, choose the most effective or principal means of control.

(A) Rat control
(B) Sanitation
(C) Immunization
(D) Vector control
(E) None of the above

406. AIDS

407. St. Louis encephalitis

408. Typhoid fever

409. Tetanus

Questions 410–413

Match the following.

(A) Hemolytic anemia in premature infants
(B) Hemorrhagic disease of the newborn
(C) Wound healing
(D) Rickets
(E) Polyneuritis

410. Vitamin C

411. Vitamin E

412. Vitamin D

413. Vitamin K

Questions 414-417

For each disease, indicate the material in which the infectious agent is transmitted from the infected host.

(A) Conjunctival exudate
(B) Lesion exudate
(C) Blood
(D) Respiratory secretions
(E) Feces

414. Syphilis

415. Shigellosis

416. Pertussis

417. Trachoma

Questions 418-421

Match each infection below with the intermediate host involved in transmission.

(A) Snail
(B) Swine
(C) Fish
(D) Crab
(E) Dog

418. Paragonimiasis (lung fluke disease)

419. Diphyllobothriasis

420. Toxocariasis (visceral larva migrans)

421. Cysticercosis

Questions 422-425

Select the reservoir for each of the diseases below.

(A) Cattle
(B) Humans
(C) Rodents
(D) Ticks
(E) Rabbits
(F) Mosquitoes
(G) None of the above

422. Candidiasis

423. Plague

424. Brucellosis

425. Enterobiasis

Primary and Secondary Prevention of Specific Illnesses

Answers

329. The answer is B. *(Last, ed 12. pp 1479-1486.)* Because of the consistent effectiveness of fluoride in reducing dental caries by about 50 percent, its use is now widely accepted among public health professionals. Controversy surrounding fluoridation is political, not scientific. The optimum concentration of fluoride in drinking water decreases with increasing mean air temperature because people drink more water when it is hotter. Moderate fluorosis occurs at a fluoride concentration of about 2 ppm; severe fluorosis at 3 ppm.

330. The answer is C. *(Last, ed 12. pp 216-218.)* Type B *Haemophilus influenzae* is by far the most virulent type and accounts for almost all cases of invasive disease. (Remember: B is for bad.) The most important of these diseases are meningitis, epiglottitis, pneumonia, and periorbital or facial cellulitis, and their occurrence is mainly in children. Previous vaccines were not effective in children under 18 months of age. However, a new vaccine made of capsular polysaccharide conjugated with diphtheria toxoid can be given to children beginning at 2 months of age. *H. influenzae* is the second most common cause of acute otitis media in children (after pneumococcus), but most cases are due to nontypable strains, rather than to type B. Because ampicillin resistance is increasingly common, life-threatening *H. influenzae* infections should be initially treated with both ampicillin and chloramphenicol, or with one of the newer cephalosporins, such as cefotaxime or ceftriaxone.

331. The answer is B. *(USPS Task Force, pp lvi-lvii, 121-124, 139-146, 201-208, 225-232.)* Universal screening for hepatitis B surface antigen (HBsAG) in pregnant women is based on evidence that early treatment of the newborn with hepatitis B immune globulin and subsequent vaccination is 85 to 95 percent effective in preventing development of the chronic carrier state in infants born to HBsAG-positive mothers. Screening only high-risk groups misses 35 to 65 percent of chronic carriers, presumably because of lack of information about maternal substance abuse and sexual habits. Since the test and treatment are both efficacious and relatively inexpensive, and there is a large at-risk population, routine screening is recommended.

In populations where hepatitis B is endemic (e.g., Alaskan natives, Pacific islanders), universal vaccination with hepatitis B vaccine may be more practical.

Currently, HIV testing is recommended only for mothers identified as high-risk, although this recommendation could change as the AIDS epidemic spreads and evidence for the efficacy of early treatment of infants increases. Hemoglobin electrophoresis is only recommended for people at high risk for sickle cell anemia or thalassemia. Ultrasound is recommended for women with either uncertain menstrual histories or risk factors for intrauterine growth retardation.

332. The answer is C. *(California Department of Health Services, California Morbidity, no. 44, 1986.)* Most patients with antibodies to HIV have the virus in their lymphocytes. Early hopes that only 10 percent of infected persons would get AIDS were overly optimistic: the risk of developing AIDS continues for years, so that the cumulative risk reaches about 30 to 40 percent in 4 years and continues to rise thereafter. The ELISA test is very sensitive and specific (both about 99 percent), but in low-risk populations, in which the prevalence of true infection may be 0.1 percent or less, the predictive value is low. False positives cannot occur in patients with AIDS because any positive result would be a true positive. False negatives do, however, occur. Antibody-negative patients can probably transmit the disease because development of antibody positivity takes a few months after exposure.

333. The answer is A. *(Whitney, ed 2. pp 414, 496, 537–538.)* For adult men and nonmenstruating women, the recommended daily dietary intake of elemental iron is 10 mg. Menstruation increases the daily needs of women to 18 mg of iron. After menopause, the iron requirement for women becomes the same as that for men. Cow's milk contains little or no iron. Because the requirement for iron is high during periods of rapid growth (as in infancy), iron-fortified milk formulas or cereals are recommended for infants. Patients with hemolytic anemias like thalassemia do not need extra iron. In fact, iron toxicity from tranfusions is a major problem in such patients.

334. The answer is A. *(Wilson, ed 12. pp 968–969.)* There is extensive evidence showing reduction of mortality among patients with coronary heart disease with the use of beta blockers among survivors of myocardial infarction, and with aspirin among patients with unstable angina as well. Nitrates and calcium channel blockers are useful for the treatment of angina, but there is no evidence they reduce mortality (nitrates have not been studied for their effects on mortality). Compared with medical therapy, coronary artery bypass grafting prolongs life in patients with left main coronary artery disease (more than a 50 percent occlusion) and those with three-vessel coronary artery disease and poor left ventricular function.

335. The answer is A. *(Whitney, ed 2. pp 427–430.)* The importance of dietary iodine rests only on its role as an essential component of thyroid hormone. The thyroid gland extracts the minute amounts of iodine in the diet for synthesis of thyroid hormone. If there is adequate iodine in the soil, plant foods (and animals that eat them) will have sufficient content of iodine. Seafood is also rich in iodine. If dietary iodine is insufficient, the thyroid gland enlarges (goiter) in order to be better able to extract the small amounts available. This generally allows the patient to remain euthyroid. The thyroid gland very avidly concentrates iodine, especially when the diet has been deficient. Because ^{131}I is a radioactive isotope present in atomic fallout, persons at risk of exposure to fallout (for example, Western Europeans after the accident at the Chernobyl nuclear reactor) may be advised to take iodide from existing (safe) supplies prior to exposure, so that if they are exposed to radioactive iodine, which has been shown to cause thyroid cancer, they will absorb less of it.

336. The answer is D. *(Benenson, ed 15. pp 200-207.)* In some areas of Southeast Asia, the prevalence of the hepatitis B carrier state is 20 percent or more. Vertical transmission from asymptomatic infected mothers to their infants is thought to be the major mode of perpetuation of the high endemic carrier rate because hepatitis B acquired in infancy is much more likely to result in chronic infection than is infection acquired later. Chronic carriers are important not only as reservoirs for hepatitis, but also because of their very high risk of hepatocellular carcinoma. For this reason it is essential to screen women for hepatitis B carriage during their pregnancy, so that the infant can be given hepatitis B immune globulin and hepatitis B vaccine, which have been shown to be 90 percent effective at interrupting vertical transmission of the disease. In the United States, the infection is primarily transmitted horizontally through exposure to blood or blood products via either needles (e.g., in drug addicts, recipients of factor VIII concentrate, hospital workers) or mucous membranes (via sexual contact). Employees of dialysis centers are among those at highest risk. The fecal-oral route is not an important route of transmission of hepatitis B, although it is for hepatitis A.

337. The answer is D. *(Centers for Disease Control, Immunization against Disease [1983], pp 72-73.)* Routine use of BCG for hospital workers is not recommended. Surveillance of personnel for newly acquired tuberculosis infection by means of routine tuberculin skin testing is preferable to BCG. Typhoid vaccination is not recommended because of the very low incidence of typhoid fever in the United States. Administration of pneumococcal vaccine to all hospital employees is not recommended; however, those who are at high risk of pneumococcal disease because of underlying medical conditions should be immunized. All female employees of childbearing age who work with pediatric patients should be vaccinated with rubella vaccine unless they have serologic proof of immunity. All personnel of both sexes, including physicians, who have direct contact with pregnant women in the hospital or clinics should have serologic testing for susceptibility to rubella performed and should be immunized if susceptible.

338.   The answer is D. *(Wilson, ed 12. p 1792.)* Most authorities believe that adding a progestin will reduce the risk of endometrial cancer associated with estrogen-only preparations. The effects on coronary heart disease, which is the leading cause of mortality in women, are the most important. Unlike oral contraceptives, there is no effect of postmenopausal hormonal replacement therapy on pulmonary embolism. There may be a slightly increased risk of breast cancer.

339.   The answer is A. *(Benenson, ed 15. pp 89–94.)* Antibiotics and oral-fluid therapy have been the major factors in reducing the case-fatality rate of cholera. Treatment of cholera with tetracycline reduces the volume and duration of diarrhea, thus reducing the need for intravenous administration of fluids. Glucose-electrolyte solutions for oral administration not only have been shown to be well absorbed and capable of maintaining fluid and electrolyte balance but also have reduced the need for intravenous fluid therapy. An effective cholera vaccine has not yet been developed. In any case, vaccination and chlorination would be expected to reduce the incidence, not the case-fatality rate.

340.   The answer is C. *(Benenson, ed 15. pp 138–142.)* Diphtheria toxoid, alone or in combination with pertussis vaccine and tetanus toxoid (DTP), induces protective levels of antitoxin that persist for about 10 years. Boosters are required every 10 years after completion of primary immunization in order to maintain protective concentration of antibody. Antitoxin antibodies do not prevent infection of the respiratory tract with *C. diphtheriae* and do not prevent the development of the carrier state. The antibodies are directed against the exotoxin produced by the bacteria, not against the bacteria themselves. Adverse reactions from the toxoid are very infrequent in infants and young children but are more common in adults; therefore, the administration of a reduced dose of toxoid is recommended for children over 6 years of age and adults. The reduced dose is symbolized by a lower case d. It is usually combined with tetanus toxoid as a Td.

341.   The answer is D. *(Benenson, ed 15. pp 474–479.)* The infectious agent for epidemic forms of typhus fever is *Rickettsia prowazecki*, which is transmitted from person to person by the human body louse, *Pediculus humanus corporis*. Disruptions of social and economic institutions by war, famine, or natural catastrophes are associated with declining standards of personal hygiene and spread of lice. Even before social and economic recovery after World War II, epidemic typhus was controlled by mass application of DDT powder. This insecticide killed the body lice; thus the transmission cycle was interrupted. Effective antibiotic therapy with chloramphenicol and tetracycline was not available until the early 1950s. *Anopheles* mosquitoes are vectors in the transmission of malaria, not typhus.

342.   The answer is A. *(Benenson, ed 15. pp 269–275.)* The injection of live attenuated measles vaccine induces protective antibodies in 95 percent of susceptible children; this seroconversion, or development of active immunity, persists for over 12 years. Postimmunization encephalitis is very rare (1 per 1 million doses) and subacute sclerosing panencephalitis has not been linked definitely to vaccine use. Leukemia and other conditions associated with immunosuppression are contraindications to the use of live measles vaccine because of the risk of developing severe or fatal giant-cell pneumonia.

343. The answer is D. *(Benenson, ed 15. pp 460-465.)* Preventive treatment is treatment of *inactive* tuberculosis—that is, tuberculosis without evidence of disease—and has as its objective the reduction of the incidence of active tuberculosis. Preventive treatment with isoniazid, or isonicotinic acid hydrazide (INH), is recommended for children and young adults whose tuberculin tests are positive, for those who have had contact with persons who have recently converted to tuberculin positivity, and for immunosuppressed persons whose tuberculin tests are positive. Because of the risk of INH-associated hepatitis, preventive treatment with INH is no longer routinely recommended for adults over age 35 and is not recommended for prevention of tuberculosis caused by atypical mycobacteria. Breast feeding is not a contraindication to INH. In a risk-benefit analysis to assess the potential effectiveness of INH, consideration should be given to the high susceptibility to infection of children under 3 years of age, of adolescents, and of young adults.

344. The answer is D. *(Benenson, ed 15. pp 199, 226-227, 294-295.)* Passive immunization is the provision of antibodies that are already formed rather than of antigens, which are used for active immunization. For example, viral hepatitis type A infection can be prevented by the administration of immune serum globulin. German measles, mumps, and influenza are best prevented by active immunization with vaccines.

345. The answer is B. *(Benenson, ed 15. pp 185-189.)* Both tetracycline 500 mg qid for a week and ampicillin 3.5 g plus probenecid 1 g taken at one time are effective in eradicating non-penicillinase-producing *Neisseria gonorrhoeae*. The single dose therapy has the advantages of improved compliance and infrequent side effects. However, because up to 45 percent of patients with gonorrhea have coexisting chlamydial infection, tetracycline should be considered, in spite of its less convenient dosage schedule and tendency to cause mild gastrointestinal discomfort. (These problems are less severe with doxycycline, but doxycycline is considerably more expensive.) In addition, many authorities recommend combining the treatments to get the benefits of both. Pregnancy is a contraindication to treatment with tetracycline because of possible effects on the developing teeth.

346. The answer is D. *(American Academy of Pediatrics, pp 429-451.)* Asymptomatic children with positive PPD skin tests should have a chest x-ray. If there are no signs of active disease, they should be treated with isoniazid (INH) 10 mg/kg per day to a maximum of 300 mg per day, for a period of at least 6 months. In low-risk patients, most tests will be negative, and the chance of tuberculosis is so small that many positive tests will be false positives caused by cross-reacting atypical myco-bacteria. For these reasons, annual testing of low-risk children is no longer recom-mended. Adults with tuberculosis are much more likely to be contagious than children. The finding of any person with tuberculosis or a recent skin test conversion mandates investigation of other members of the household.

347. The answer is B. *(Cherry, Pediatrics 81:939-984, 1988.)* Common adverse reactions after pertussis vaccine include fever, irritability, and significant local reac-tions in approximately half of the recipients. The frequency of these side effects is reduced significantly by administration of 10 to 15 mg/kg of acetaminophen at the time of vaccination and 4 h later. High fever (41°C [105.8°F]) occurs in 1 to 2 percent of children. Brief grand mal seizures occur at a rate of approximately 1/1,750 injections. Vasomotor collapse characterized by pallor and lethargy occurs at a similar rate. Hypoglycemia resulting from the stimulation of insulin released by the vaccine has been reported. Prolonged crying occurs in 5 percent of children. The risk of permanent brain damage is estimated from the British Childhood Encepha-lopathy Study to be approximately 1/310,000, although more recent studies ques-tion this association.

348. The answer is C. *(Benenson, ed 15. pp 200-207.)* Hepatitis B virus (HBV) infection has an incubation period of 6 weeks to 6 months, compared with 2 to 6 weeks for infections caused by hepatitis A virus (HAV). Specific diagnosis of HBV infection can be made by the detection of hepatitis B surface antigen (HBsAg) in the blood during the acute stage of the infection or by detecting antibodies to a variety of antigens of HBV in the convalescent stage. HBsAg may persist in the blood for many years: the chronic carrier state develops in 10 percent of HBV infections in adults. Chronic carriage of HBsAg is associated with a significantly increased risk of chronic hepatitis, cirrhosis, and hepatocellular carcinoma. Hepatitis B immune globulin (HBIG), a preparation of immune globulin containing high titers of anti-HBs, is an effective means of preventing infection if administered within 72 h after exposure to HBV. Vaccines made from either highly purified HBsAg derived from plasma of healthy chronic carriers or from HBsAg produced by genetically engi-neered bacteria have been shown to be highly effective in preventing HBV infection. Administration of HBIG followed by three doses of vaccine is 90 percent effective in preventing vertical (mother-to-baby) transmission.

349. The answer is A. *(Benenson, ed 15. pp 66-68.)* Prevention of human brucel-losis depends on pasteurization of dairy products from cows, goats, and sheep; education of farmers and workers in the livestock industry as to dangers of infected animals; and care in handling products from aborted animals. There is no insect vector. No vaccine for human use is available. Since person-to-person transmission does not occur, treatment of individual cases will not control spread of brucellosis.

350. The answer is C. *(Benenson, ed 15. pp 224–228.)* Influenza vaccine is not recommended for routine use in the entire population because current vaccines produce immunity lasting only 1 to 2 years and are only 60 to 70 percent effective. Periodic changes in the viral antigens also contribute to absence of long-term efficacy of vaccines. High-risk groups include all persons over 65 years of age, persons with chronic heart and lung conditions, and persons with other chronic diseases such as diabetes, neuromuscular disorders, and renal failure. Pregnant women have not been shown to be at increased risk of excess morbidity or mortality during recent epidemics. Routine immunization of school children is not recommended with the current vaccines even though school-age children are the major age group involved in the transmission of influenza in the community. If safe, effective vaccines with long-lasting immunity are developed, school children will be the major target group.

351. The answer is D. *(Benenson, ed 15. pp 61–66.)* Botulism is an intoxication by the exotoxin produced by *Clostridium botulinum*, a gram-positive, spore-forming bacterium. The incubation period is usually 12 to 36 h. In the United States, most cases are associated with ingestion of improperly home-canned vegetables, fish, and fruits, especially foods that are slightly acidic. The toxin is destroyed by boiling for at least 3 min, but higher temperatures are needed to kill the spores. At inadequate temperatures, spores are not destroyed; they subsequently germinate and multiply under anaerobic conditions. Death is usually the consequence of respiratory paralysis or secondary infection. An antitoxin is available and is considered part of routine treatment.

352. The answer is D. *(Last, ed 12. pp 190–192.)* HSV-2, the main cause of genital herpes, is currently epidemic in the U.S. Many infections are asymptomatic, which makes it difficult to prevent further spread. Infants acquire the infection from their mothers during vaginal delivery; for mothers with known active HSV-2 infections, caesarian delivery within 4 h of rupture of membranes is indicated. HSV-2 infection is not an early sign of AIDS—unlike infections such as *Pneumocystis carinii*, its occurrence does not suggest immunosuppression. Neonates with any signs of HSV infection should receive antiviral therapy; one of the goals is to prevent dissemination.

353. The answer is C. *(Rudolph, ed 18. pp 519–521, 547.)* The pertussis vaccine is associated with relatively frequent side effects, probably because it is a concentrated suspension of whole, killed pertussis bacteria, rather than a toxoid. There is no placental transfer of immunity to pertussis, so immunization is begun as soon as the infant is able to mount any kind of response—2 months of age (with diphtheria and tetanus toxoids) is the current recommendation. Immunity is not developed until after the second injection and lasts only a few years. Thus adults, although they do not develop the classic whopping cough picture, are very often susceptible to pertussis. Protection against diphtheria and tetanus is afforded by immunization with toxoids. Patients who have completed their primary immunization series and have had a booster in the last 5 years are not at risk for tetanus and require neither tetanus immune globulin nor additional tetanus toxoid. Those who need additional tetanus toxoid should get a Td to maintain their immunity to diphtheria.

354.   The answer is C. *(Last, ed 12. p 412.)* Infection of hogs with nematodes of the genus *Trichinella* can be prevented by ensuring that all garbage and offal fed to the hogs are heat-treated to destroy the cysts or, preferably, by using feed devoid of animal meat, such as grain. Prohibition of marketing of garbage-fed hogs is easier to enforce than inspection to ensure that all garbage is properly cooked. Thorough cooking of pork and pork products so that all the meat reaches at least 58.3°C (137°F) destroys the encysted larvae. Freezing pork also destroys the larvae if adequate time-temperature schedules are followed. The disease is transmitted by ingestion of larvae in skeletal muscle, not by hog feces.

355.   The answer is D. *(Benenson, ed 15. pp 255-257.)* Lyme disease is caused by a spirochete, *Borrelia burgdorferi*, transmitted to humans by the bite of infected ticks. The name comes from the town (Old Lyme, Connecticut) from which the first cases were reported. There are endemic foci on the east coast from Massachusetts to Virginia, and in Wisconsin, Minnesota, California, and Oregon. The hallmark of the disease is the characteristic rash, which begins as a red papule (usually at the site of the tick bite) and slowly spreads outward in an advancing annular fashion. This lesion is called erythema chronicum migrans (ECM). Subsequently, joints (either acute or chronic arthritis), CNS (an aseptic meningitis or encephalitis), and heart (atrioventricular arrhythmias or myopericarditis) may be involved. These complications may be diminished by early treatment with tetracycline or penicillin.

356.   The answer is D. *(Benenson, ed 15. pp 31-32, 257-259, 280-284.)* Meningococcal disease is transmitted by direct contact with droplets and discharges from infected cases and, more often, carriers. California encephalitis and St. Louis encephalitis are acute, inflammatory diseases in which the causative virus is mosquito-transmitted. Lymphocytic choriomeningitis is caused by an arenavirus acquired from contact with food or dust contaminated with urine, saliva, and feces of infected mice. Person-to-person transmission does not occur in these last three diseases.

357.   The answer is E. *(Wilson, ed 12. pp 1585-1586.)* The efficacy of exfoliative cytology (Pap smear) in early identification of uterine and cervical cancer has been demonstrated. Mortality from cervical cancer has consistently declined following screening programs based on the Pap smear. Current recommendations are to perform the test every 3 years following three normal Pap smears in consecutive years.

358. The answer is B. *(Wilson, ed 12. pp 995-996.)* The most important preventable risk factors for coronary artery disease (CAD) are hypercholesterolemia (especially an elevated LDL level), cigarette smoking, and hypertension. Of these three risk factors, however, evidence from randomized trials showing a reduction in CAD is available only for treatment of elevated cholesterol levels. An elevated HDL level is associated with a reduced risk of CAD. The death rate from ischemic heart disease is five times higher in white men ages 35 to 55 compared with white women of the same age.

359. The answer is A. *(Wyngaarden, ed 18. pp 292-293.)* Treating hypertension can reduce the incidence of stroke by up to 90 percent. Most persons with hypertension in the U.S. (70 percent) are aware of their condition. Treatment of hypertension appears to be equally efficacious in men and in women.

360. The answer is E. *(Last, ed 12. pp 1151-1155.)* The purpose of a cancer screening technique is to detect the disease at an asymptomatic phase. This is helpful only if early treatment is more effective than later treatment. Detection of lung cancer with radiography in asymptomatic smokers does not meet this requirement.

361. The answer is B. *(Expert Panel, Arch Intern Med 148:37-69, 1988.)* Serum cholesterol is carried on three major types of molecules: low-density lipoproteins (LDLs), high-density lipoproteins (HDLs), and very-low-density lipoproteins (VLDLs). VLDLs are mostly triglycerides; the amount of cholesterol carried on VLDL is approximated as the triglycerides divided by 5. LDL cholesterol is difficult to measure and thus is usually estimated indirectly by the following formula:

$$\text{LDL cholesterol} = \text{Total cholesterol} - \text{HDL cholesterol} - \text{triglycerides}/5$$

In this example, LDL = $300 - 40 - 200/5 = 220$ mg/dL. This is considered to be a very elevated LDL cholesterol (normal is less than 130 mg/dL). Note that the formula is not valid when the triglycerides are greater than about 400 mg/dL.

362. The answer is E. *(Wilson, ed 12. p 998.)* Many patients with hypercholesterolemia can lower their plasma cholesterol levels by reducing the intake of total calories, saturated fat, cholesterol, and alcohol; however, dietary changes, unless they are severe, do not usually lower plasma cholesterol levels by more than 10 to 20 percent. In low-to-moderate quantities (about two drinks per day) alcohol increases the high-density lipoprotein levels (i.e., has a beneficial effect), whereas at higher doses it increases low-density lipoprotein levels (i.e., has a harmful effect). Vitamin E levels in serum are affected by lipid levels; however, the reverse is not true.

363.   The answer is A. *(Wyngaarden, ed 18. pp 1444–1445.)* Postmenopausal estrogens (PME) are commonly prescribed for the relief of menopausal symptoms (such as hot flashes) and for the prevention of postmenopausal osteoporosis. They do appear, however, to increase the incidence of endometrial cancer by about three to five times. Fortunately, this is a rare disease (incidence of about 1/100,000), and nearly all PME-associated endometerial cancers have been seen at early stages (perhaps because of an earlier presentation with estrogen-induced postmenopausal bleeding). Recently, some have advocated adding progestins to PME regimens to decrease the risk of endometrial cancer. However, the progestins may negate the beneficial effects of PME on serum lipids (estrogens raise HDL levels) and thus reduce the benefits of PME on coronary heart disease. Recent studies have suggested that PME may be associated with perhaps a 50 percent increase in incidence of breast cancer.

364.   The answer is B. *(Wyngaarden, ed 18. pp 292–293.)* Contrary to common belief, systolic hypertension is as strong a risk factor for cardiovascular disease as is diastolic hypertension. Isolated systolic hypertension (ISH) is defined as a systolic pressure greater than 160 mmHg with a normal diastolic pressure (<90 mmHg). The prevalence of ISH increases with age in both men and women.

365.   The answer is C. *(Wilson, ed 12. pp 1268–1281.)* Both types of inflammatory bowel disease are more common in whites than blacks and Asians. Jews have three to six times the incidence of non-Jews. There is no sex preference. The peak incidence of both diseases occurs between the ages of 15 and 35. There is an increased risk of colonic malignancy associated with ulcerative colitis, especially among those with pancolitis, who have a risk of cancer of about 40 percent after 24 years of the disease. However, prophylactic colectomy is no longer routine. Instead, periodic colonoscopy with biopsy of suspicious areas is recommended. Patients with pancolitis associated with Crohn's disease are at a slightly increased risk of colonic malignancy and should also have periodic colonoscopy.

366.   The answer is C. *(Wilson, ed 12. p 967.)* Prognosis is related to the type and severity of coronary artery stenosis and the quality of the function of the left ventricle. Critical stenosis of the left main coronary artery, for example, is associated with a mortality of about 15 percent each year. The severity of myocardial ischemia (as reflected by angina or a markedly positive exercise test) is also predictive. Family history of heart disease is a risk factor for the incidence of coronary artery disease. Such a history, however, has not proved to be a predictor of prognosis for the disease. Elevated serum cholesterol levels, on the other hand, are associated with increased mortality following myocardial infarction. Treatment has been shown to be beneficial.

367.   The answer is A. *(Last, ed 12. pp 598–599.)* Although most lead intake in humans is from ingestion of lead-contaminated food—about 0.3 mg of lead is ingested daily per person—the amount of lead that is absorbed after inhalation of lead-contaminated air is of greater significance because up to 50 percent of inhaled lead, compared with only as much as 10 percent of ingested lead, is absorbed and circulated by the blood. Because modern building codes usually require the replacement of lead domestic water-supply pipes by those made of copper or galvanized iron, drinking water has become a decreasing source of lead poisoning. The intake of lead through ingestion of lead-based paint is mainly a problem in children.

368.   The answer is D. *(Rosenstock, pp 1–3.)* Occupational diseases are an important health problem in the U.S. Their diagnosis remains a challenge, partly because the presentations of these diseases are usually not distinguishable from those unrelated to occupational exposures. In addition, there may be a lengthy interval between the occupational exposure and the first manifestations of the disease, and clinicians may not ascertain the nature of those exposures. Although certain occupational exposures, such as those to coal and silica dust, are associated with chronic obstructive pulmonary disease, cigarette smoking is responsible for about 90 percent of all deaths due to the disease in the U.S.

369.   The answer is D. *(Last, ed 12. pp 1278–1279.)* Once a back injury has been sustained, the muscles and ligaments of the injured areas are weaker than before the injury. Mechanical lifting devices should be used so that unassisted lifting can be avoided. Accident prevention programs should include consideration of a worker's physical condition and age as well as the frequency with which strenuous work is part of the work schedule. Back injuries often occur when workers do not readjust their grasp on a heavy, bulky load after it has been lifted. Preemployment radiographs are not helpful.

370.   The answer is B. *(Last, ed 12. pp 503, 901.)* More than 15,000 chemicals are used by industries, but threshold limit values (TLVs) exist for about 500 of them. Existing TLVs have been established on the basis of average exposures; thus, during the performance of a certain task, workers may be exposed at times to unhealthy levels of a toxic chemical. Furthermore, TLVs were established without consideration of the interaction of industrial chemicals and of the cumulative effect of exposure to these chemicals. The regulatory agencies have limited personnel resources and thus are unable to determine the degree of industrial compliance with all regulations.

371. The answer is E. *(Croog, N Engl J Med 314:1657–1664, 1986. Wyngaarden, ed 18. p 289.)* Almost all drug-induced depression responds to discontinuing the drug. The prevalence is highest in patients using centrally active drugs, such as reserpine, methyldopa, and beta blockers; up to 30 percent of such patients report symptoms compatible with depression. Although drug-induced depression can exacerbate underlying depression, it is most often seen in people who are psychologically healthy. There is no relationship between the prevalence of depression and the degree of lowering of blood pressure.

372. The answer is A. *(Kaplan, ed 5. pp 686–698, 1743.)* The fetal alcohol syndrome occurs in infants born to mothers who drink frequently and heavily during the pregnancy. Abnormalities in such infants include mental retardation, increase in perinatal mortality, microcephaly, short palpebral fissures, midfacial defects, abnormal hands and feet, ventricular septal defects, and hemangiomas. About 2 live births per 100,000 have the complete syndrome. Recent work suggests that occasional alcohol consumption during pregnancy does not substantially affect the fetus.

373. The answer is B. *(Last, ed 12. pp 1519–1520.)* Kwashiorkor results from a diet that is severely deficient in proteins and often sufficient or slightly deficient in calories. It occurs in toddlers after their weaning from breast milk to a diet high in carbohydrates and low in proteins and is characterized by changes in hair texture and color, ulcerated skin lesions, hepatomegaly, edema secondary to hypoalbuminemia, diarrhea, impaired liver function, and apathy.

374. The answer is D. *(Last, ed 12. p 1023.)* Nicotine-containing chewing gum is a useful adjunct in helping smokers to quit. It is most successful in smokers who report high levels of addiction, but should be used in the context of a comprehensive program for cessation of smoking. Each stick of gum contains about 2 mg of nicotine, roughly the equivalent of one cigarette.

375. The answer is A. *(Kaplan, ed 5. pp 599–641.)* In the United States today, organic brain syndrome from syphilis or vitamin B deficiency is an unusual occurrence. (In the early 1900s, syphilis and vitamin deficiency were leading causes for admissions to mental hospitals.) However, many chemical agents, including lead and alcohol, are still causes of organic brain syndrome.

376–379. The answers are: 376-C, 377-E, 378-B, 379-A. *(Last, ed 12. pp 1520–1524.)* Scurvy due to *vitamin C deficiency* is characterized by pain and tenderness of the extremities, irritability, and hemorrhagic phenomena, all the result of defective formation of collagen. *Niacin deficiency* causes pellagra, which results in the four D's: disturbances of the gastrointestinal tract (*d*iarrhea), of the skin (*d*ermatitis), and of the nervous system (*d*elirium and *d*ementia). *Thiamine deficiency* leads to beriberi in which either myocardial disease (edema and cardiac failure) or neurologic signs predominate. *Vitamin A deficiency* leads to defects in epithelial cells of skin (hyperkeratosis) and to eye disorders (xerosis and keratomalacia, as well as night blindness). *Vitamin D deficiency* causes rickets in children and osteomalacia in adults; both conditions are due to the inadequate mineralization of bone.

380–384.   The answers are: 380-B, 381-B, 382-D, 383-A, 384-D. *(USPS Task Force, pp xlii–xlix. Hoekelman, pp 22–23.)* In the birth-to-18-month-old age group, leading causes of death include conditions originating in the perinatal period, congenital anomalies, infections, and nonmotor vehicle injuries (i.e., injuries not involving a motor vehicle). Routine blood testing is recommended in this age group as part of the neonatal screen, which may include screens for phenylketonuria, galactosemia, hypothyroidism, and hemoglobinopathies. (At all other ages, only high-risk patients should have blood tests performed.) Growth and development are monitored regularly. Counseling of parents should include nutrition, injury prevention, dental health, and effects of passive smoking. Routine immunization and chemoprophylaxis include ophthalmic antibiotics and diphtheria-pertussis-tetanus (DPT), measles-mumps-rubella (MMR), polio, and *Haemophilus influenzae* vaccines.

In the 2-to-6-year-old age group leading causes of death are injuries (nonmotor vehicle more often than motor vehicle), congenital anomalies, neoplasms, and homicide. Growth and development continues to be monitored and initial blood pressure measurements begin. Counseling includes exercise, dental hygiene, and diet with an emphasis on caloric balance. Dental visits begin. Injury prevention is again stressed and bicycle safety helmets recommended. Polio and DPT boosters are given at 4 to 6 years.

In the 7-to-12-year-old age group leading causes of death include injuries (motor vehicle more often than nonmotor vehicle), neoplasms, congenital anomalies, and homicide. Growth, development, and blood pressure continue to be monitored. Diet, exercise, injury prevention, and dental health continue to be reviewed and appropriate patient and parent counseling performed. A measles booster is recommended at entry into either elementary or middle school.

In the 13-to-18-year-old age group leading causes of death include motor vehicle crashes, homicide, suicide, nonmotor vehicle injuries, and cancer. Historical information is gathered and counseling given about diet, exercise, substance use, risk-taking behaviors, emotional well-being, and sexual practices. Given the importance of suicide in this age group, the history should include screening for stresses such as family difficulties, school problems, depression, and substance abuse. The physical examination should include cultures in sexually active adolescents. A tetanus-diphtheria booster (Td) is given at 14 to 16 years and every 10 years thereafter. Pertussis vaccination is not indicated in people over 7 years of age.

385-388.   The answers are: 385-B, 386-D, 387-C, 388-A. *(Benenson, ed 15. pp 50-52, 219-221, 418-420, 427-429, 450-451.)* *Necator americanus*, the American hookworm, enters the skin (usually of the foot) in the larval stage. The larvae are carried via lymphatics and blood to the lungs, where they migrate up the airways to be swallowed. They reach maturity and begin laying eggs in the intestine in 6 to 7 weeks. Autoinfection does not occur because the eggs are not infective for 7 to 10 days. Hookworm disease is primarily due to iron deficiency anemia from chronic gastrointestinal blood loss.

The life cycle of *Ascaris lumbricoides* begins when a person ingests infectious eggs. In the intestine these hatch into larvae, which migrate through the portal circulation to the lungs. After that, the life cycle is similar to that of *Necator americanus*: migration through the alveoli to airways, swallowing, and maturation and laying of eggs in the intestine. *Ascaris* eggs also are not immediately infectious; they require about 2 weeks of incubation. Thus ascariasis is also not directly transmissible from person to person.

The life cycle of *Strongyloides stercoralis* is similar to that of hookworm: larvae enter the skin, travel to the lungs, ascend the trachea, are swallowed, and develop into mature, egg-laying worms in the intestine. However, a crucial difference is that the eggs of *Strongyloides* may develop into infective filariform larvae even before leaving the host, and these larvae may pass through the perianal skin, leading to autoinfection and increasing worm burden. This occurs most often in immunocompromised patients.

Taenia solium, the pork tapeworm, is acquired by ingestion of inadequately cooked pork that is infected with taenia cysticerci ("measly pork"). The cysticerci develop into egg-laying adult tapeworms in the intestine. However, unlike those of the beef tapeworm (*Taenia saginata*), eggs of *Taenia solium* are infective to humans. The ingested eggs develop into larvae, which then migrate throughout the soft tissues of the body, including the brain, eye, and heart.

Trichuris trichiura, or whipworm, has a relatively simple life cycle: after embryonated eggs are ingested, they develop into larvae, then adult worms. The worms lay eggs that are not infectious for at least 3 weeks; thus, person-to-person transmission and autoinfection do not occur.

389-392.   The answers are: 389-C, 390-B, 391-E, 392-A. *(Benenson, ed 15. pp 255-257, 316-318, 364-366, 385-388, 474-477.)* *Sarcoptes scabiei* is the name of the mite that causes scabies. The disease is due to the inflammatory response to the mite, which burrows under the skin and deposits eggs and feces. Treatment is with gamma benzene hexachloride (lindane; Kwell).

Pediculus humanus capitis, the head louse, causes epidemics among school children and institutionalized patients. A preparation of 1% permethrin (a synthetic pyrethrin) is the treatment of choice; lindane is a slightly less effective alternative.

Pediculus humanus corporis, the body louse, is the only louse that is an important vector of disease. It is the vector for epidemic typhus and relapsing fever, as well as for trench fever. It is most closely associated with severe poverty and lack of cleanliness.

Lyme disease is caused by a spirochete, *Borrelia burgdorferi,* transmitted to humans by infected ticks. The incubation period ranges from 3 days to a month after exposure; treatment is with tetracycline (in adults) or penicillin (in children).

393–396. The answers are: 393-D, 394-E, 395-B, 396-A. *(Whitney, ed 2. pp 420–427, 430–431, 433–435.)* Chromium is found in food in several different complexes, including a small organic molecule called *glucose tolerance factor,* which seems to be important for normal carbohydrate metabolism. Deficiency of chromium impairs the action of insulin, and a diabetes-like condition ensues.

Cobalt's main function in the body is as a part of vitamin B_{12}, which is also called *cobalamine.* Deficiency syndromes linked to cobalt are those associated with deficiency of the vitamin. Chronic administration of cobalt can lead to goiter as a result of blocking iodine uptake by the thyroid.

Selenium is a component of glutathione peroxidase, an enzyme that works with vitamin E to protect cells from oxidative damage. The growth of human fibroblasts and other cells in tissue culture requires selenium. The metal cures or prevents Keshan disease, which is characterized by multifocal myocardial necrosis and is endemic to Keshan Province in China.

Zinc is involved with many metabolic pathways, including those responsible for healing of wounds, sexual development, and taste. Developing fetuses, pregnant women, and growing children have higher requirements for zinc than do adult men and nonpregnant women.

Copper is important for formation of red cells and collagen and for the function of the central nervous system.

397–401. The answers are: 397-B, 398-A, 399-E, 400-B, 401-C. *(Wilson, ed 12. p 24.)* Screening programs for genetic diseases should be targeted at the ethnic or racial groups at highest risk. Blacks, for example, are at an increased risk of sickle cell disease. This includes both hemoglobin S and hemoglobin C. Blacks also have a higher incidence of other hemoglobinopathies, including both alpha and beta thalassemia. They also have a higher risk of glucose-6-phosphate dehydrogenase (G6PD) deficiency. G6PD deficiency is also seen in Chinese and Mediterranean people. Persons from the Mediterranean (including Greeks, Italians, and Sephardic Jews) are also at risk of familial Mediterranean fever and beta thalassemia. The Chinese are at increased risk of alpha thalassemia. Ashkenazic Jews (from Poland and Russia) are at increased risk of a variety of genetic diseases, including Tay-Sachs disease and Gaucher disease. Northern Europeans are at risk of cystic fibrosis. Alpha₁-antitrypsin deficiency is especially frequent in Scandinavians. Porphyria variegata is more common in whites from South Africa. Hemophilia is seen in all ethnic groups.

402–405. The answers are: 402-C, 403-E, 404-C, 405-A. *(Friedland, N Engl J Med 317:1125–1135, 1987. Hearst, JAMA 259:2428–2432, 1988.)* Although we are in the midst of a monstrous AIDS epidemic, it is important to know that the disease is less infectious than many sexually transmitted diseases. The chance of acquiring the virus depends on the infectivity of the virus and the probability that the contact is infected.

The infectivity from a single episode of penile-vaginal intercourse is very roughly estimated to be about 1/500. (The infectivity is probably higher for anal intercourse and is higher for vaginal intercourse in the presence of genital ulcers.) Condoms are estimated to reduce the risk of transmission by about 90 percent. This reduction is relatively small compared with the effect of selection of a sexual partner. The prevalence of infection in men not belonging to any high-risk group is estimated at roughly 1/10,000, compared with 1/20 to 1/2 in men belonging to a high-risk group. Thus the risk of HIV from a single sexual encounter with a man not at high risk is about 1/500 × 1/10,000, or 1/5,000,000. The risk from 10 such encounters is approximately 10 times as high, or 1/500,000, still much less than 1/100,000.

The risk of transmission from infected blood depends largely on the size of the inoculum. Two-thirds of blood recipients from infected donors seroconvert, compared with only 1/100 to 1/1,000 persons exposed by accidental needle-sticks or exposures to mucous membrane.

406–409. The answers are: 406-E, 407-D, 408-B, 409-C. *(Benenson, ed 15. pp 1–7, 31–35, 430–433, 469–474.)* The principal means of controlling the AIDS epidemic is to effect reductions in high-risk behavior. Both antibody testing (to identify persons capable of transmitting the infection) and education (to inform people of which behaviors are most unsafe) are important components of such efforts. In addition, careful screening of donors, testing of the blood supply, and heat treatment of factor VIII concentrates have reduced transmission of the infection through blood products.

St. Louis encephalitis is caused by a virus in the flavivirus family, one of a group of *ar*thropod-*bo*rne ("arbo") viruses. The disease is transmitted by the bite of an infected mosquito. The viruses are difficult to culture; the diagnosis is generally suspected clinically and confirmed serologically. Control of the arboviral encephalitides requires control of the insect vector—in this instance elimination of breeding grounds for mosquitos, destruction of larvae, screening of sleeping and living quarters, and application of residual insecticides.

Unlike other species of salmonella, *Salmonella typhi*, the cause of typhoid fever, is found only in human beings; there is no animal reservoir. *S. typhi* is excreted in the feces of human carriers. Therefore, control of the disease primarily requires adequate sanitation. Sporadic cases continue to occur in the U.S.; these should be investigated by public health authorities, and the actual or probable source of the infection should be identified.

Immunization with tetanus toxoid is the best means of protection against tetanus. Since the causative organism is a normal inhabitant of the intestine of many animals (including human beings), the need for immunization will persist in spite of the present rarity of the disease. Persons who have sustained dirty wounds should receive tetanus immune globulin (TIG) unless they have an up-to-date status of tetanus vaccination (three past doses of tetanus toxoid, the most recent within the past 5 years).

410–413. The answers are: 410-C, 411-A, 412-D, 413-B. *(Last, ed 12. pp 1520–1524. Rudolph, ed 18. p 1053.)* Vitamin C is necessary for normal collagen formation. Lack of vitamin C inhibits wound healing as well as causes scurvy. Numerous claims (each lacking substantiation) of benefits from vitamin E supplements have been made, including prevention of abortion, prevention of coronary heart disease, and improvement of lactation. One of the few demonstrated vitamin E deficiency states is a hemolytic anemia that occurs in premature babies. Rickets results from inadequate vitamin D intake leading to failure of absorption of calcium and phosphate. Hemorrhagic disease of the newborn due to low levels of prothrombin and of other clotting factors can be prevented by administration of vitamin K_1 immediately after birth.

414–417. The answers are: 414-B, 415-E, 416-D, 417-A. *(Benenson, ed 15. pp 320, 392, 422, 443.)* Infectious agents have developed a variety of means of transmission from one host to the next. Syphilis is spread by direct contact with exudates from early lesions of the skin or mucous membranes, or both of these, usually during sexual activity. Such lesions usually contain large numbers of spirochetes. Infection by indirect contact with contaminated objects rarely occurs because of the lack of viability of the organisms outside the body.

During the diarrheal stage of shigellosis, large numbers of bacteria are excreted. The infectious dose for humans is as low as 100 bacteria; thus the disease is highly contagious, especially among young children who practice poor personal hygiene. Poor sanitation that allows contamination of food or water can cause large scale outbreaks.

Pertussis, on the other hand, is transmitted in the respiratory secretions of infected persons during talking, coughing, sneezing, or singing. Direct person-to-person spread results from inhaling droplets containing the bacteria. Children are most contagious during the initial (catarrhal) stage, during which large numbers of bacteria are present in the profuse nasal secretions. The number of bacteria present in respiratory secretions falls rapidly during the second (paroxysmal) stage of the disease.

Trachoma, a chronic infection of the conjunctiva, is caused by *Chlamydia trachomatis* and is spread by contact with infected discharges from the eye. Direct person-to-person spread is the major means of transmission, although indirect mechanical transmission by flies may also occur. Trachoma is one of the major preventable causes of blindness in the world.

418–421.   The answers are: 418-D, 419-C, 420-E, 421-B. *(Benenson, ed 15. pp 142-144, 314-316, 427-429, 435-437. Last, ed 12. p 411.)* Paragonimiasis is caused by the lung fluke, *Paragonimus westermani*. It has a complex life cycle in which larval stages undergo development in fresh-water crabs and other crustacea. Infection occurs by eating infected raw crabs. The disease, which affects the lungs, causing chronic cough and hemoptysis, occurs primarily in the Far East but has recently been reported in the western hemisphere.

Diphyllobothriasis is the disease caused by the fish tapeworm, *Diphyllobothrium latum*, which uses fresh-water fish as its intermediate host. One or two percent of infections are complicated by megaloblastic anemia caused by interference with vitamin B_{12} absorption or by competition between the worm and the host for dietary vitamin B_{12}.

Toxocariasis is caused by the dog roundworm, *Toxocara canis*. The disease occurs mainly in children as the result of ingestion of soil contaminated with *Toxocara* eggs. Development of the *Toxocara* is incomplete in humans so that the larval stages migrate through the body—hence the term *visceral larva migrans*.

Cysticercosis is caused by the pork tapeworm, *Taenia solium*. Intestinal infection occurs by eating pork infested by cysts of *T. solium*. The adult tapeworm resides in the intestinal tract from which gravid proglottids (segments containing eggs) are shed in the feces. If the eggs hatch in the intestinal tract, the larvae can migrate throughout the body, often reaching the brain. Cysticercosis is a common cause of epilepsy in Mexico and other third-world countries.

422–425.   The answers are: 422-B, 423-C, 424-A, 425-B.   *(Benenson, ed 15. pp 67, 73, 157, 325.)* The reservoir of *Candida albicans* is the human gastrointestinal tract. Candidal organisms, frequently part of the normal flora in the human body, cause disease only when host defenses are impaired as a result of disease, drug treatment, or altered immune response.

Numerous species of wild rodents are the natural reservoir of plague, in which transmission is through the bites of fleas infected with *Yersinia pestis*. While control of urban plague has been achieved in most of the world, plague still exists in rural areas of the United States, South America, Africa, and the Middle East, and in Central and Southeast Asia. The potential of spread from the wild rodent reservoir to domestic rats, and then to humans, still exists.

Cattle, pigs, sheep, horses, reindeer, and goats are the main reservoirs of brucellosis. A systemic disease in humans, brucellosis may be acquired from raw milk or cheese from infected animals. It is also an occupational disease of farmers, abattoir workers, veterinarians, and others who have contact with animals that may be infected. Important economic losses can be caused by brucellosis in domestic animals.

Enterobiasis is an intestinal infection with the pinworm, *Enterobius vermicularis*. The most common symptom is anal itching, particularly at night. There is no animal reservoir, but infective eggs may survive in household dust for up to 2 weeks; hence careful daily sweeping or vacuuming for a few days after treatment may prevent reinfestation.

Provision of Health Services

DIRECTIONS: Each question below contains five suggested responses. Select the **one best** response to each question.

426. Which of the following statements concerning maternal and child health (MCH) programs is correct?

(A) The Women, Infants, and Children (WIC) program provides low-cost preventive health care services to women and their children
(B) All children living at or below the poverty level are eligible for Medicaid
(C) Crippled children's services must be provided by the states, under Title V of the Social Security Act
(D) Funds for MCH programs remained stable under the Reagan administration
(E) None of the above

427. Which of the following health measures has the greatest potential for prevention of disease in the U.S.?

(A) Environmental modification
(B) Genetic counseling
(C) Immunization
(D) Modification of personal health behavior
(E) Screening tests

428. Which statement about Medicare is correct?

(A) Reimbursements are made to persons over 60 years of age for certain health care expenditures
(B) Reimbursements are made to persons listed on state welfare roles for certain health care expenditures regardless of age
(C) Reimbursement for hospitalization is based on diagnosis-related groups
(D) The program covers complete hospitalization costs for eligible persons
(E) None of the above

429. Guidelines for effective patient education and counseling include all the following EXCEPT

(A) obtaining commitment from patients to change behavior
(B) involving office staff
(C) involving patients in selection of risk factors that require change
(D) using a single strategy
(E) monitoring progress through follow-up contact

430. All the following statements about the resource-based Relative Value Scale (RVS) are correct EXCEPT

(A) its purpose is to allow more equitable reimbursement of hospitals based on the cost of producing specific services
(B) it will lead to increasing reimbursement for primary care
(C) it will lead to decreased reimbursement for most surgery
(D) the proposed fees are similar to those already in place in Canada
(E) proponents hope that it will increase the incentive for physicians to spend more time with patients

431. Following a nuclear war, survivors would be threatened by both increased frequency and increased lethality of infectious diseases. Which of the following factors would increase the *lethality* of infections?

(A) Crowding in shelters
(B) Dramatic increase in the insect population
(C) Immunosuppressive effects of fall-out radiation
(D) Destruction of sanitation systems
(E) None of the above

432. Principal findings of the United States Preventive Services (USPS) Task Force include all the following EXCEPT

(A) acute care visits are an appropriate setting for preventive services
(B) interventions that address personal health behavior are among the most effective
(C) more data and research are necessary to assess the effectiveness of various preventive services
(D) patients must assume greater responsibility for their own health
(E) screening tests should be applied uniformly

433. What percentage of total expenditures for health care in the U.S. is paid by private health insurance?

(A) 16 percent
(B) 32 percent
(C) 47 percent
(D) 61 percent
(E) 75 percent

434. Payments for personal health expenditures can be grouped into two categories: (1) direct payments, made out-of-pocket by the individual; and (2) third-party payments, made by insurance companies, government-sponsored programs, or philanthropic agencies. True statements concerning sources of payment of personal health expenditures in the United States include which of the following?

(A) Government payments, as a percentage of the total, have more than doubled since 1940
(B) Direct payments constitute 50 percent of the total
(C) Health insurance payments, as a percentage of the total, have stayed constant since 1950
(D) Blue Cross covers over half of all persons insured for personal health expenditures
(E) None of the above

435. Health care expenditures in the United States have increased from $12.7 billion in 1950 to $539.9 billion in 1988. About what proportion of the gross national product was spent on health care in 1988?

(A) 2 percent
(B) 6 percent
(C) 11 percent
(D) 15 percent
(E) 20 percent

436. Appropriate considerations for implementation of a screening test include all the following EXCEPT

(A) burden of suffering
(B) cost of screening test
(C) the physician's familiarity with the disease
(D) potential adverse effects of screening test
(E) efficacy of treatment

437. Physicians often fail to provide preventive medical services for all the following reasons EXCEPT

(A) insufficient financial reimbursement for preventive services
(B) insufficient time with patients during routine visits
(C) lack of published guidelines for routine care
(D) lack of routine visits by patients for health care maintenance
(E) uncertainty as to which services should be offered

438. Which of the following categories of service accounted for the largest proportion of health care costs in the United States in 1984?

(A) Physicians
(B) Hospitals
(C) Drugs
(D) Nursing homes
(E) Dentists

439. In 1988, $539.9 billion was spent on health in the United States. Approximately what proportion was devoted to (noncommercial) medical research?

(A) 2 percent
(B) 4 percent
(C) 6 percent
(D) 8 percent
(E) 10 percent

440. All the following comparisons of the U.S. and Canadian health care systems are true EXCEPT

(A) the percentage of the GNP devoted to health care is higher in the U.S.
(B) the percentage of people who are uninsured is higher in the U.S.
(C) quantity of physician services per capita is higher in the U.S.
(D) fees for physician services are higher in the U.S.
(E) net incomes of physicians are higher in the U.S.

441. All the following statements comparing uninsured working-age adults to insured adults are true EXCEPT that uninsured adults

(A) are more likely to be poor, young, and unmarried
(B) are less likely overall to have contact with a health care provider
(C) have fewer ambulatory visits per year
(D) have lower out-of-pocket medical expenses
(E) are more likely to receive their care in an emergency room or hospital clinic

442. Correct statements regarding casualties from nuclear war include all the following EXCEPT

(A) in the immediate postattack period, casualties due to blast and thermal injuries would predominate
(B) long-term atmospheric effects ("nuclear winter") would be more severe if the attack occurred in July than in January
(C) a limited (100-megaton) attack on 100 U.S. cities would result in about 15,000,000 to 50,000,000 immediate deaths
(D) a major (6,500-megaton) nuclear attack on the U.S. would result in few if any (less than 1 million) immediate survivors
(E) in a major nuclear war, millions of casualties in noncombatant countries would be expected

443. Which of the following statements about graduates of foreign (non-U.S.) medical schools is correct?

(A) Most foreign medical graduates in residency training in the U.S. are not U.S. citizens
(B) Foreign medical graduates account for about one-third of physicians in residency training in the U.S.
(C) About one-fifth of U.S. physicians are foreign medical graduates
(D) Less than half of foreign medical graduates are involved in direct patient care
(E) None of the above

444. All the following statements concerning reported legal abortions are true EXCEPT

(A) the number of legal abortions has progressively decreased since 1980
(B) the number of abortions per 1,000 live births is higher among minority women
(C) the number of abortions per 1,000 live births is higher among women less than 15 years of age
(D) most abortions are performed during the first trimester
(E) women undergoing legal abortion tend to have no previous live births

445. All the following statements concerning diagnosis-related groups (DRGs) are correct EXCEPT

(A) they are the basis for prospective payment for Medicare patients
(B) patients are assigned to DRGs based on information from hospital discharge abstracts
(C) reimbursement for patient care provided is the same in different communities, and for teaching and nonteaching hospitals
(D) a problem with DRG-based reimbursement is that it provides a financial incentive to increase admissions of patients who are less ill
(E) DRGs have resulted in substantial reductions in Medicare expenditures

446. In 1988, the highest infant mortality was reported for

(A) Canada
(B) East Germany
(C) Spain
(D) Singapore
(E) United States

447. All the following are reasons for rapidly rising malpractice premiums EXCEPT

(A) investment losses by carriers of liability insurance
(B) payments of awards in installments rather than lump sums
(C) increased numbers of claims filed by plaintiffs
(D) increased size of malpractice awards
(E) the fact that new medical technologies raised expectations

448. True statements about maternal age and total fertility in the United States in 1987 include all the following EXCEPT

(A) births to women under age 15 were increasing
(B) birth rates for women ages 15 to 30 had remained unchanged for several years
(C) birth rates for women over age 30 were increasing
(D) total fertility rates were higher for blacks than for whites
(E) the overall total fertility rate was above the replacement level

449. In analysis of cost-effectiveness, health benefits and costs that will not occur until some time in the future are often less highly valued. This process is called

(A) depreciation
(B) amortization
(C) discounting
(D) cost-shifting
(E) none of the above

450. Which of the following statements regarding for-profit health care in the U.S. is correct?

(A) Psychiatric hospitals and nursing homes are much more often operated for profit than are general hospitals
(B) For-profit hospitals generally have lower costs than nonprofit hospitals
(C) After peaking in the late 1970s, the number of proprietary (for-profit) hospitals in the U.S. is decreasing
(D) Indicators of quality of hospital care, such as board certification of staff physicians and outcome of elective surgery, have generally shown that investor-owned chain hospitals are slightly superior to nonprofit or public hospitals
(E) None of the above

451. The world population is currently estimated to be growing at a rate such that the time required for the population to double is

(A) 15 years
(B) 35 years
(C) 70 years
(D) 105 years
(E) 140 years

452. An analysis of cost-effectiveness discloses that hemodialysis for a 50-year-old patient costs about $30,000 to $35,000 per quality-adjusted year of life (QALY) saved. This indicates that

(A) hemodialysis is not cost-effective
(B) hemodialysis results in a relative low quality of life
(C) placing a patient with renal failure on dialysis increases his or her life expectancy
(D) the annual incremental cost of hemodialysis is more than $40,000
(E) life expectancy of a patient on hemodialysis is less than 20 years

453. The number of Americans with no health insurance coverage is approximately

(A) 1,000,000
(B) 15,000,000
(C) 30,000,000
(D) 45,000,000
(E) 60,000,000

454. Correct statements about nursing home care in the U.S. include all the following EXCEPT

(A) mental or behavioral problems are present in the majority of nursing home residents
(B) the mean age of nursing home patients is 70 years
(C) about 20 percent of the population over age 85 are in nursing homes
(D) white women are the most frequent inpatients in nursing homes
(E) more than half of expenses for nursing home care is paid from public funds

455. Statements that correctly characterize the operations of the Medicaid program include which of the following?

(A) Payments are made to providers of specified health care services for specified groups of low-income people
(B) Benefits are provided to recipients who meet eligibility criteria that have been determined principally at the federal level
(C) Funding does not depend on individual state contributions
(D) Program administration is primarily the responsibility of the Social Security Administration
(E) None of the above

456. All the following were recommendations of the Bipartisan Commission on Comprehensive Health Care (the "Pepper Commission") EXCEPT

(A) tax subsidies to small employers to subsidize health insurance
(B) prohibition of exclusions from health insurance for "pre-existing conditions"
(C) public insurance coverage for the poor and unemployed
(D) nationwide standards for minimum benefits
(E) gradual phasing-in of a Canadian-style single-payor system over the next 10 years

457. Which of the following factors contributed to the increase in hospital costs over the past 10 years in the United States?

(A) Increased length of stay
(B) Increased competition among hospitals
(C) Increased numbers of hospital admissions
(D) Increased use of high-technology modes of diagnosis and treatment
(E) None of the above

458. True statements about the relationship between socioeconomic status and psychiatric hospitalization include all the following EXCEPT

(A) the ratio of hospitalized to non-hospitalized psychotic patients is higher in lower- than in upper-class families
(B) upper-class families are greatly reluctant to use state hospitals
(C) upper-class families are less likely to care for patients at home
(D) upper-class families make greater use of nursing homes
(E) the incidence of psychosis is greater in lower-class families

DIRECTIONS: Each group of questions below consists of lettered headings followed by a set of numbered items. For each numbered item select the **one** lettered heading with which it is **most** closely associated. Each lettered heading may be used **once, more than once, or not at all.**

Questions 459–462

Match each description below to the proper health care organization.

(A) Professional Review Organization (PRO)
(B) Health Maintenance Organization (HMO)
(C) Independent Practice Association (IPA)
(D) Preferred Provider Organization (PPO)
(E) None of the above

459. Nonprofit association of physicians that reviews the quality of care provided to Medicare, Medicaid, and other patients

460. Group of providers that agree to provide services to specific groups of patients on a discounted fee-for-service basis

461. An organization that directly provides or arranges for all health services required by a defined population of prepaid clients

462. An organization that contracts with private physicians in the community to provide services to members of prepaid group health plans

Questions 463–466

For each function or program select the responsible agency.

(A) Food and Drug Administration
(B) Department of Agriculture
(C) Centers for Disease Control
(D) National Center for Health Statistics
(E) Environmental Protection Agency

463. Immunization and health education

464. Standards for drug manufacture

465. Guidelines of solid waste management

466. Women, Infants, and Children (WIC) food assistance program

Questions 467–470

Match each of the following.

(A) A private voluntary health agency
(B) A federal health agency
(C) A professional health organization
(D) An international health agency
(E) A health foundation

467. American Public Health Association

468. American Cancer Society

469. Pan American Health Organization

470. Centers for Disease Control

Provision of Health Services

Answers

426.   The answer is C. *(Last, ed 12. pp 1709-1717. Rudolph, ed 18. p 2. Williams, ed 3. pp 118-119.)* The Women, Infants, and Children (WIC) program provides food *vouchers* (not health services) for pregnant and nursing women and children up to age 5. Eligibility is based on income (<85 percent of the poverty level in 1983). Funds for crippled children are administered through the states, with matching funds through the federal government, under Title V of the Social Security Act. Funding for maternal and child health was cut (by about 20 percent) by the Reagan administration, including funding for family planning, which is among the most cost-effective of public health programs. Medicaid is the largest public funding source for medical care for children in the United States, but eligibility is limited and varies from state to state. Currently, only about half of U.S. families living at or below the poverty level are eligible for Medicaid, although recent legislation will gradually expand eligibility to all poor children.

427.   The answer is D. *(USPS Task Force, pp xx-xxii.)* Although environmental modification, genetic counseling, immunization, and screening tests are important elements of preventive health, changing personal health behavior has the largest potential for improving public health in the United States, where the leading causes of death include heart disease, cancer, AIDS, injuries, and chronic obstructive pulmonary disease. Thus, alterations in personal health behaviors—such as smoking, diet, exercise, use of seatbelts, and safe sexual behavior—need to be stressed. Priorities would be different in third-world countries where infectious disease and malnutrition are leading causes of death.

428.   The answer is C. *(Last, ed 12. pp 1657-1658.)* Medicare provides reimbursement for certain health care expenditures for persons 65 years of age and over. People less than 65 *on dialysis* are also covered. Administration of the program is primarily the responsibility of the Social Security Administration. Providers of inpatient care are reimbursed based on which of 468 diagnosis-related groups (DRGs) best fits the patient's reason for hospitalization. Program coverage for hospitalization is not complete: the patient must pay a set amount per hospitalization (the deductible).

429. The answer is D. *(USPS Task Force, pp lix–lxi.)* One should use a combination of strategies in counseling patients for maximum effectiveness rather than relying on a single strategy. Individual counseling can be supplemented with classroom instruction, support groups, written material, and audiovisual aids. However, these materials are not a substitute for individual attention and feedback. Other principles for effective counseling in addition to those listed include counseling all patients, developing a therapeutic alliance with patients, ensuring that patients understand the relationship between health and behavior, working with patients to evaluate obstacles to behavioral change, developing a behavioral modification program, involving office staff in promotion of behavioral change, and clinician role-modeling of health-promotion behaviors.

430. The answer is A. *(Wilson, ed 12. p 12.)* The resource-based Relative Value Scale (RVS) is a system for making *doctor's fees* more equitable—it does not address hospital reimbursement. It is meant to replace the "usual and customary rate" (UCR) schedule, which strongly rewarded technical procedures at the expense of cognitive services. For example, under the RVS, the physician reimbursement for repair of an inguinal hernia would decrease from $503 to $233, and that for a coronary artery bypass (three grafts) from $3,652 to $1,936, while that for a limited office visit would increase from $19 all the way to $24. (That's equity.) Proponents hope that the scale will discourage overuse of procedures and encourage physicians to spend more time with patients.

431. The answer is C. *(Abrams, N Engl J Med 305:1226–1232, 1981.)* Among many other factors, lack of medical personnel and supplies and decreased host defenses related to radiation-induced immunosuppression would increase the lethality of infectious diseases after a nuclear war. Many other factors, including lack of sanitation, increases in insect vectors, millions of corpses awaiting disposal, crowding in shelters, and disease spread from domestic and wild animals will increase the spread of disease but have much less effect on the lethality of disease.

432. The answer is E. *(USPS Task Force, pp xix–xxiii.)* The USPS Task Force was a 4-year, multidisciplinary, systematic effort to evaluate various preventive health measures. The task force published a book containing its assessment of 169 interventions in three different areas: screening, counseling, and immunization/chemoprophylaxis. The main finding was that personal health behavior (e.g., smoking, diet, exercise) is a major contributor to mortality and disability. The task force stressed the role of the physician as educator and counselor in addressing these behaviors while giving patients more responsibility for their own health. Other principal findings emphasized the need for greater *selectivity* in the application of screening tests, that is, careful consideration of the patient's age, sex, and other individual risk factors before applying screening tests. Evaluation of the screening tests revealed a need for better data to assess accurately the efficacy and appropriate frequency of the various measures. Additionally, since many patients only contact health care professionals for acute problems, the task force recommended including preventive health measures in illness visits for people with limited access to or inclination toward medical care.

433. The answer is B. *(Office of National Cost Estimates, Health Care Financing Rev 11:1-41, 1990.)* In 1988, 32 percent of all U.S. health expenses were paid by benefits from private health insurance policies. Direct payments by patients covered 21 percent of expenditures for health care and philanthropic or charitable sources 5 percent. The remaining 42 percent came from public (government) programs.

434. The answer is A. *(Office of National Cost Estimates, Health Care Financing Rev 11:1-41, 1990.)* Government payments (from federal, state, and local funding sources) composed 16 percent of total personal health expenditures in 1940 and 42 percent in 1988. According to recent tabulations by the Health Care Financing Administration, direct payments constituted 21 percent of the $2,124 per capita cost of personal health care in 1988. Health insurance payments as a percentage of the total have more than tripled from about 9 percent in 1950 to about 32 percent in 1988.

435. The answer is C. *(Office of National Cost Estimates, Health Care Financing Rev 11:1-41, 1990.)* The percentage of the gross national product spent on health care increased from 4.6 percent in 1950 to 11.1 percent in 1988. This amounts to approximately $2,124 per person. About 47 percent of these expenditures were for institutional (hospital and nursing home) care, and 19 percent for physician services.

436. The answer is C. *(USPS Task Force, pp xxvii-xxxiii.)* A variety of factors need to be considered before instituting any preventive health measure, including a screening test. The burden of suffering includes both the severity and the prevalence of the disease. Other things being equal, rare diseases are less important than more common diseases, and illnesses of minor clinical significance less important than illnesses with high morbidity and mortality. Recall also that the positive predictive value of a screening test increases as prevalence of the disease increases. Another requirement for the rational institution of a screening program is the availability (both technically and socioeconomically) of effective treatment. If no effective intervention is available for a disease, screening will only serve to produce a lead-time bias: an apparent prolongation of life by detecting a disease at an earlier stage without a true impact on survival. Additional criteria for screening tests include cost, efficacy, and potential adverse effects. The ideal screening test is inexpensive and reliable (high sensitivity and specificity). Low specificity and prevalence lead to many patients with false positive results, who must then undergo further evaluation and therapy with the attendant risk of iatrogenic morbidity. The targeting of screening tests to populations specifically at risk rather than to the population as a whole will limit costs, reduce the number of false positives, and hence decrease the adverse effects of screening.

A physician's familiarity with a disease is not an important consideration when compared with the above criteria. Primary care physicians can screen for quite uncommon diseases with which they are unfamiliar (e.g., galactosemia) as long as they know where to refer patients who test positive. As medical science progresses, screening tests offer a means of educating both practitioner and patient.

437.   The answer is C. *(USPS Task Force, pp xx–xxi.)* A variety of factors enter into an overall lack of preventive medical services. Many Americans are uninsured or underinsured, have no regular medical provider, and seek care only in urgent situations. These people do not have routine visits for health care maintenance. For these people the acute care visit is an important setting for the delivery of preventive health services because it may be their only contact with health care professionals. Furthermore, preventive services are poorly reimbursed compared with more invasive services. This financial disincentive, combined with time pressures during routine visits, discourages physicians from providing preventive measures such as investigation of health behavior risk factors and counseling. Paradoxically, more invasive and financially rewarding measures may be encouraged, such as treadmill testing, which, while appropriate to high-risk populations, should not be applied to the general population.

Physicians interested in preventive health measures may be uncertain as to which measures to institute. There is no lack of published guidelines for preventive health; recommendations are available from a variety of sources including professional and volunteer organizations as well as scientific and governmental bodies. Other sources of physician uncertainty may include skepticism of the efficacy of preventive measures and concerns of subjecting an asymptomatic, healthy person to possibly harmful interventions.

438.   The answer is B. *(Office of National Cost Estimates, Health Care Financing Rev 11:1–41, 1990.)* Hospital costs accounted for 39 percent of national health expenditures in the United States in 1988, more than twice as much as costs of physician services (19 percent). The proportions of total health care costs devoted to nursing homes, drugs, and dentists were 8, 7, and 7 percent, respectively.

439.   The answer is A. *(Office of National Cost Estimates, Health Care Financing Rev 11:1–41, 1990.)* Of the national health expenditures in 1988, 1.83 percent went to medical research, a total of $9.9 billion. The proportion expended on research had been only 0.9 percent in 1950. Following the establishment of the National Institutes of Health and the expansion of federal funding of research, the proportion of health care dollars going to research increased dramatically, reaching a peak of 3.6 percent in 1965. Currently the federal government funds approximately 80 percent of noncommercial research. Commercial research expenditures were over $5 billion in 1988.

440. The answer is C. *(Fuchs, N Engl J Med 323:884-890, 1990.)* Despite greater expenditures per capita and in percentage of GNP on health care in the U.S., a greater percentage of Americans are uninsured and lack access to medical care. The difference in expenditures is especially remarkable in terms of physician services. In 1985, physician expenditures per capita were $347 in the U.S. and $202 in Canada. This difference is entirely explained by higher fees; physician services per capita are actually lower in the U.S. than in Canada. Physician fees for diagnosis and management are approximately 80 percent higher in the United States; fees for procedures are approximately triple Canadian fees. However, net incomes of physicians are only about a third higher in the U.S., perhaps because of higher overhead and lower workload.

441. The answer is D. *(Freeman, Health Serv Res 24:811-823, 1990.)* Estimates of the country's uninsured persons range from 10 to 18 percent of the general population; adding the underinsured increases this even further. Among working-age adults, the uninsured are more likely to be young, poor or near-poor, unemployed, and unmarried. They have fewer ambulatory visits, are less likely to see a medical provider overall, and when seen tend to receive care episodically in emergency rooms or in hospital clinics. Although they receive less medical care, out-of-pocket expenses are higher. These differences are not explained on the basis of health status—the uninsured are not healthier than the insured. One goal of universal health insurance is to help correct these inequities.

442. The answer is D. *(Abrams, N Engl J Med 305:1226-1232, 1981. Daugherty, pp 207-232.)* Most deaths in the period immediately after a nuclear attack would be due to blast effects (e.g., the pressure from the blast knocking down buildings) and thermal effects (burns from intense heat generated by the explosion and from resultant fires). Estimates of immediate deaths range from around 20,000,000 from a "limited" (100-megaton) war to about 90,000,000 from a large (6,500-megaton) exchange. Note that 1 megaton is equivalent to about 80 Hiroshima bombs. Immediate casualties, however, could easily be dwarfed by longer-term problems with infection, famine, radiation, and ecologic effects. The ecologic effects depend on many factors, including the numbers and sizes of fires, deposition of their smoke, and season of the year. Nuclear winter effects would be much more severe in the summer because there would be less rain and snow to bring soot back to earth and because cooling of the earth's surface relative to normal temperatures would be much greater. Noncombatant countries, particularly those in the third world, would suffer millions of casualties related to loss of food, fertilizer, medicines, and other essential items previously provided by the United States and other countries.

443.   The answer is C. *(Igelhart, N Engl J Med 313:831-836, 1985.)* In 1983 the AMA estimated that about 21 percent of the nation's physicians were foreign medical graduates, and about 80 percent of these physicians were involved in patient care. In 1985 there were 13,451 foreign medical graduates in U.S. residency training; of these, 7,386 (55 percent) were American citizens. Overall, 18 percent of physicians in accredited residencies in 1985 were foreign medical graduates, but there was enormous variability from state to state: New Jersey (59.5 percent) and New York (37.9 percent) had the highest proportion of foreign medical graduates in their residency programs.

444.   The answer is A. *(Koonin, MMWR CDC Surveill Summ 39:23-56, 1990.)* The number of legal abortions reported to the CDC has been relatively stable over the past decade at 1.3 million per year. The abortion ratio, the number of abortions per 1,000 live births, was 356/1,000 in 1986 and was higher among minority women and women less than 15 years old. The abortion rate, the number of abortions performed per 1,000 women of childbearing age (defined as 15 to 44), was 24/1,000 per year in 1987. Women undergoing legal abortions tended to be young, white, and unmarried. They also tended to have had no previous live births and to be undergoing the procedure for the first time. Approximately half of all abortions were performed within the first 8 weeks of gestation, and 85 percent within the first trimester. Future Supreme Court decisions may affect the availability of legal abortions.

445.   The answer is C. *(Igelhart, N Engl J Med 314:1460-1464, 1986. Stern, N Engl J Med 312:621-627, 1985.)* Diagnosis-related groups (DRGs) became the basis for Medicare reimbursement October 1, 1983, following passage of the Tax Equity and Fiscal Responsibility Act of 1982, which called for Medicare to develop a prospective payment system. Patients are assigned to DRGs based on hospital discharge abstracts, and the hospital receives a fixed level of compensation for certain DRGs. The compensation does vary somewhat from hospital to hospital, depending on wage costs in the community and whether the hospital is a teaching hospital, since teaching hospitals tend to care for sicker and more indigent patients. A potential problem with DRG-based reimbursement is that, because reimbursement is based only on the DRG, the hospital will make much more profit from hospitalizing patients with marginal indications for hospitalization. A possible benefit of DRGs is increased specialization of hospitals, so that hospitals will selectively provide the services they can provide most efficiently. Provision of services at low cost, however, depends not only on efficiency but also on case mix. Thus, distinguishing between specialization and "skimming" (selection of patients who will be least expensive to care for) may be difficult. DRGs have resulted in substantial cost savings: along with other cuts they have resulted in cost savings of about $40 billion between 1981 and 1986. While defense spending increased under the Reagan administration from 22 to 26 percent of the budget, Medicare declined from 7.6 to 7.1 percent.

446. The answer is E. *(Wegman, Pediatrics 84:943–957, 1989.)* In 1987 the United States tied with Italy for 21st place worldwide in infant mortality, with 10.1 deaths per 1,000 live births. Japan ranked first (5.0) with provisional rates for 1988 even lower. Other countries ranking above the United States include Canada (7.3), Singapore (7.4), East Germany (8.5), and Spain (8.5). These comparisons also hold true if one only considers infant mortality for whites in the United States (8.6). Advocates for stronger prenatal care use these data to illustrate the inadequacies of the delivery system for health care in the United States.

447. The answer is B. *(LeMasurier, Health Care Financing Rev 7:111–116, 1985.)* Malpractice insurance premiums increased by 221 percent between 1975 and 1984, compared with a 107 percent increase in the consumer price index. There is considerable debate about the relative importance of investment losses and losses from paid claims, but numbers of claims and sizes of verdicts have been increasing. Payment of awards in installments, rather than in lump sums, has resulted in savings of up to 14 percent rather than increased costs to the insurance industry.

448. The answer is E. *(Wegman, Pediatrics 84:943–956, 1989.)* The total fertility rate is calculated by applying the age-specific rates through a woman's childbearing years. A total fertility rate of 2,110 per 1,000 women (or 2.11 per woman) will lead to zero net population growth in the absence of in- or out-migration. In 1987 the overall U.S. rate was 1.87, a 2 percent increase from 1986. Total fertility rate for black women was 2.29 compared with 1.77 for white women. Age-specific birth rates (the number of births per year per 1,000 women in the specified age group) in the United States in 1987 reflect an increase in birth rates to women above age 30, with the greatest percentage increase occurring in women ages 35 to 39. In contrast the birth rate for women ages 15 to 30 has remained essentially constant for several years. However, at the lower end of the scale, total births to women under age 15 increased by 1 percent in 1987, and the birth rate for women ages 15 to 19 also increased.

449. The answer is C. *(Wilson, ed 12. p 13.)* Discounting is the term used to describe the reduced value of costs and benefits first realized in the future. It is dependent on monetary inflation, as well as on the extent to which society wishes to invest today's dollars for future health. Depreciation and amortization refer to the process by which capital investments are written off over a period of years. Cost-shifting occurs when the costs of care for some people (usually poor and uninsured) are shifted to others who are able to pay the bills.

450.   The answer is A. *(Gray, N Engl J Med 314:1523-1528, 1986. Relman, N Engl J Med 303:963-970, 1980.)* For-profit health care in the U.S. has been increasing dramatically in the last 10 years, expanding from nursing homes and psychiatric hospitals, which traditionally have been more frequently proprietary, to general hospitals. Clinical laboratories, home care, and hemodialysis centers are also substantially for-profit industries. For-profit hospitals do not generally have lower costs than nonprofit hospitals, but collections per case from third party payers have been 15 to 20 percent higher in for-profit hospitals. Indicators of quality of care have not shown much difference between investor-owned hospital chains and nonprofit hospitals, although historical problems with proprietary nursing homes suggest that continued caution is indicated regarding quality of care in for-profit hospitals.

451.   The answer is B. *(Mausner, ed 2. p 250.)* The population of the world grew from an estimated two billion in 1930 to four billion in 1975. The United Nations projected in 1975 that the population will double again in 35 years, reaching a total of eight billion by 2010. However, the impact of birth control programs in China and other nations may alter this estimate.

452.   The answer is C. *(Wilson, ed 12. pp 5-11.)* Hemodialysis must increase life expectancy, otherwise it would result in a situation in which there is cost per year of life lost. Quality-adjusted life years (QALYs) are an attempt to compare the value of life with a chronic medical problem (like the need for hemodialysis) with perfect health, which is assigned a value of 1.0; the quality adjustment for patients on hemodialysis would differ among patients, but would be less than 1.0—perhaps, say, 0.9. In its most simple formulation, cost per QALY saved is simply cost divided by the quality adjustment. Thus cost is cost-effectiveness times the quality adjustment, and the cost of hemodialysis (since the quality adjustment is less than 1.0) must be less than $30,000 to $35,000 per year. There is no way to determine life expectancy or quality of life in this situation, nor can one ever say whether a technology is cost-effective unless one asks against what its cost-effectiveness is to be compared.

453.   The answer is C. *(Rockefeller, N Engl J Med 323:1005-1007, 1990.)* Approximately 31,000,000 Americans have no health insurance at all. Tens of millions more are underinsured, often with hefty deductibles and copayments or coverage only for inpatient acute services. Even those who have insurance face losing it if they change their employment.

454.   The answer is B. *(Last, ed 12. pp 1331-1335, 1650-1651.)* Mental and behavioral problems are the most common conditions among nursing home patients, with senility or chronic brain syndrome occurring in about 57 percent of patients. About 20 percent of the population over 85 live in nursing homes. The mean age of all nursing home patients is over 80 years, with only 10 percent less than age 65. White women are most likely to become patients in nursing homes because they have greater longevity than blacks and males. About 65 percent of nursing home expenses come from public funds, primarily Medicaid.

455. The answer is A. *(Last, ed 12. p 1659.)* Medicaid provides federal funds on a matching basis to states that elect to enter the program. Criteria for eligibility to receive benefits and for the range of the medical services provided by the program are primarily determined at the state rather than federal level. Although legislative authority for Medicaid is derived from Title XIX of the Social Security Act, most program operations are carried out by state-employed administrators. States may impose copayments for optional services or for patients who are "medically needy" but have some resources.

456. The answer is E. *(Rockefeller, N Engl J Med 323:1004-1007, 1990.)* The Bipartisan Commission on Comprehensive Health Care ("Pepper Commission") was created by an act of Congress in 1988 to provide recommendations on reform of health care financing. The recommendations, released in 1990, are aimed at reducing some of the inequity of the current system without major changes in its structure. Financing of health care would remain primarily job-based with a tax subsidy to small employers. Insurers would be prohibited from many current practices by which they compete for patients who are "good risks," including exclusions for preexisting conditions. A minimum benefit package under federal standards would include coverage for primary care, preventive care, and catastrophic illness and would be available to the poor and uninsured. The Pepper Commission did not recommend transition to a Canadian-style system.

457. The answer is D. *(Williams, ed 3. pp 189-191.)* Over the past 10 years there has been increasing use of x-rays, laboratory tests, and high-technology therapy. The increase in costs has occurred despite a leveling off of hospital admissions and shorter hospital stays. Some of the increase, ironically, is due to the cost of complying with regulations whose goal was containment of costs.

458. The answer is C. *(Kaplan, ed 5. pp 299-307.)* Members of upper-class families often attempt to keep their relatives who have psychoses out of mental (especially public) hospitals and usually have the economic means and strong motivations to obtain home nursing care or the services of nursing homes for their relatives. The incidence of mental illness is inversely related to the level of social class.

459-462. The answers are: 459-A, 460-D, 461-B, 462-C. *(Mayer, N Engl J Med 312:590-594, 1985. Williams, ed 3. pp 144-147, 365, 395.)* Review of the quality of care is the purview of Professional Review Organizations (PROs), formerly called Professional Standards Review Organizations, which were established in the

1972 Social Security Amendments. PROs may contract with businesses as well as with the Department of Health and Human Services (DHHS) to monitor quality of care and hospital utilization.

Preferred Provider Organizations (PPOs) are groups of providers that make special arrangements with insurers to provide services to their customers on a discounted basis, i.e., to accept lower levels of reimbursement than their usual rates. An example is the Blue Cross "Prudent Buyer Plan," in which patients who are willing to obtain care from preferred providers can save on coinsurance and deductibles.

Health Maintenance Organizations (HMOs) provide comprehensive health care services on a prepaid basis. First developed around the turn of the century, they were bitterly opposed by organized medicine. In the early 1970s, legislation encouraging their development was passed, which led to the establishment of 166 HMOs by 1975 and to 323 HMOs covering 15 million members by 1985.

Independent Practice Associations (IPAs) are a more recent development. Whereas HMOs have traditionally served their patients by employing full-time physicians in their own clinics and medical centers, IPAs allow private physicians to contract with HMOs to provide services to enrolled patients.

463–466.   The answers are: 463-C, 464-A, 465-E, 466-B. *(Green, ed 6. pp 120, 441–442, 444, 455–459.)* The Centers for Disease Control's responsibilities are to provide surveillance and investigation of epidemic diseases, to promote disease-control programs, to provide expert laboratory assistance to state and local health departments, and to promote immunization and health education programs.

The Food and Drug Administration (FDA) was established in 1906 to enforce the laws that regulated interstate transport and quality of drugs and food. The FDA, which received its current name in 1931, assures that safe and effective prescription drugs are sold to the public. To do this, the FDA tests products, sets standards for production and quality control, and judges claims of safety and efficacy.

The Environmental Protection Agency (EPA) is responsible for protection and promotion of environmental quality. The EPA sets guidelines for solid waste disposal, for hazardous waste control, for recovery of resources from wastes, and for the screening of potentially hazardous chemicals prior to production and distribution.

The Women, Infants, and Children (WIC) food assistance program is the largest federally funded state health program. It is administered by the U.S. Department of Agriculture and provides supplemental food for pregnant and nursing women, infants, and children.

467–470.   The answers are: 467-C, 468-A, 469-D, 470-B. *(Green, ed 6. pp 456–459, 465, 470–471, 528.)* Professional health organizations are groups formed by persons who have met prescribed standards of training and certification and whose purposes are to promote the interests of the profession and to serve the public. An example is the American Public Health Association, founded in 1872, which establishes standards and guidelines related to public health; implements public health education through its journal, other publications, and meetings; and provides expert testimony to legislative groups.

The American Cancer Society, founded in 1913, is an example of a nonprofit, voluntary health agency, which was organized to disseminate knowledge about cancer and is supported by voluntary donations.

The Pan American Health Organization, established in 1901, is an international health agency representing the nations of the Americas. Its major concern has been control of communicable diseases. It has been integrated into the World Health Organization and serves as the regional office for the Americas.

The Centers for Disease Control, formerly known as the Communicable Disease Center, is a branch of the United States Public Health Service. It is the federal agency responsible for surveillance of communicable diseases in the United States.

Legal and Ethical Issues

DIRECTIONS: Each question below contains four or five suggested responses. Select the **one best** response to each question.

471. All the following findings should raise the suspicion of child abuse EXCEPT

(A) multiple circular scars of approximately 1 cm
(B) spiral fractures
(C) fractures of the femur in children not yet walking
(D) multiple bruises of different ages over the shins
(E) retinal hemorrhages

472. Which of the following statements regarding domestic battering of women is correct?

(A) Most instances of spouse abuse occur as isolated incidents
(B) Among married women, less than 2 percent are beaten by their husbands over the course of a year
(C) The majority of instances of woman battering are caused by alcohol abuse
(D) Presenting complaints among abused women seeking medical attention are often nonspecific
(E) None of the above

473. In order for children to enter school, all 50 states in the United States require proof of immunization against all the following infections EXCEPT

(A) measles
(B) poliomyelitis
(C) diphtheria
(D) rubella
(E) mumps

474. According to the report form (U.S. Standard Report of Fetal Death) recommended by the National Center for Health Statistics, facts required in completing a report of a fetal death include all the following EXCEPT

(A) cause of death
(B) results of autopsy
(C) weight of fetus
(D) the month in the pregnancy when prenatal care began
(E) complications of labor

475. Which of the following statements regarding informed consent for medical treatment is correct?

(A) Physicians must disclose risks of a specific treatment, but are not required to discuss alternative treatments if they are less effective
(B) Because risks of procedures may be frightening, it is best to defer the discussion until after the patient has been sedated
(C) In order to be valid, informed consent must be written and include the patient's signature and the date
(D) The primary factor in the physician's responsibility to inform the patient of an adverse effect is the frequency of that effect
(E) None of the above

476. Cholera and plague are reportable diseases according to the 1969 International Health Regulations. Other reportable diseases include all the following EXCEPT

(A) hepatitis B
(B) malaria
(C) paralytic poliomyelitis
(D) yellow fever
(E) smallpox

477. The carelessness or dereliction of duty by a professional person is called

(A) criminal negligence
(B) malfeasance
(C) misfeasance
(D) malpractice
(E) none of the above

478. In order for a patient to recover damages due to negligence, each of the following elements must be present EXCEPT

(A) duty to care
(B) breach of duty
(C) injury
(D) nonfeasance
(E) proximate cause

479. All the following statements about Good Samaritan laws are true EXCEPT

(A) they have been enacted by most states
(B) they are designed to encourage health professionals to provide assistance in emergency situations
(C) they free providers from liability for gross or criminal negligence
(D) they generally require that assistance be rendered without payment or expectation of payment for services
(E) they may apply to both professionals and laypersons

480. When debating whether providing or withholding medical treatment is ethical, the LEAST important consideration of those listed below is

(A) indications for medical intervention
(B) expected quality of life
(C) patient's preferences
(D) physician's preferences
(E) economic factors

481. As organ transplantation has become more common, guidelines have been developed to govern organ donation. The Uniform Anatomical Gift Act does all the following EXCEPT

(A) allow partial donation
(B) free health care personnel from civil and criminal liability when acting in good faith
(C) limit which physicians may certify time of death
(D) provide for revoking of a donation
(E) require express, documented consent by the donor

482. Which of the following patients is incompetent and should receive medical care against his or her expressed wishes?

(A) A 32-year-old Jehovah's Witness who had refused transfusions for a ruptured ectopic pregnancy and is now unresponsive postoperatively with a hematocrit of 8 percent
(B) An anxious, frightened 48 year old who refuses surgery for gastric cancer because "it's too scary"
(C) A 55-year-old executive with chest pain and ECG changes who refuses hospitalization because of "an important business deal"
(D) An active 83-year-old diabetic who refuses treatment for a gangrenous foot ulcer because "I'm going to die anyway"
(E) None of the above

483. All the following criteria may be the basis for withholding medical treatment in an infant with Down's syndrome EXCEPT

(A) chronic and irreversible coma
(B) parental preference
(C) treatment that merely prolongs dying but does not correct the underlying condition
(D) treatment that is futile in terms of survival

484. Physicians have obligations to report all the following EXCEPT

(A) accidental gunshot wounds
(B) births and deaths
(C) certain communicable diseases
(D) child abuse
(E) substance abuse

485. The Hippocratic Oath specifically includes all the following elements EXCEPT

(A) respect for and commitment to teachers
(B) proscriptions against abortion
(C) proscriptions against euthanasia
(D) proscriptions against sexual misconduct
(E) proscriptions against substance abuse

486. All the following principles are among the Department of Health and Human Services (DHHS) guidelines for ethical research EXCEPT

(A) confidentiality is adequately protected
(B) informed consent is obtained if appropriate
(C) subjects are adequately compensated for time or pain
(D) data are monitored to ensure safety of subjects
(E) additional safeguards are instituted for vulnerable patients

487. A physician fills out a death certificate as follows:

Immediate cause of death—
pulmonary embolism
Due to—deep venous thrombosis
Due to—pancreatic cancer

She notes that a liver biopsy was performed prior to death. In the U.S. vital statistics, this death would be recorded as due to

(A) pulmonary embolism
(B) deep venous thrombosis
(C) pancreatic cancer
(D) Trousseau's syndrome
(E) complication of liver biopsy

488. One of your patients who has metastatic breast cancer develops shortness of breath. She presents to the emergency department, where you diagnose pericarditis, which is confirmed by echocardiography. Soon after, cardiac tamponade occurs and she develops ventricular tachycardia and then ventricular fibrillation. Cardiopulmonary resuscitation is unsuccessful. Despite your request, her family refuses an autopsy. How should you indicate the cause of death on the death certificate for this woman?

(A) Cardiopulmonary arrest due to ventricular fibrillation due to ventricular tachycardia
(B) Ventricular fibrillation due to cardiac tamponade due to pericarditis
(C) Pericarditis
(D) Breast cancer
(E) The death certificate should not be filled out; this is a coroner's case

DIRECTIONS: Each group of questions below consists of lettered headings followed by a set of numbered items. For each numbered item select the **one** lettered heading with which it is **most** closely associated. Each lettered heading may be used **once, more than once, or not at all.**

Questions 489–491

Match each of the following legal cases with the relevant subject matter.

(A) Abortion
(B) Duty to warn
(C) Informed consent
(D) Malpractice liability
(E) Termination of life support

489. *Darling v. Charleston Community Memorial Hospital*

490. *In re Quinlan*

491. *Tarasoff v. Regents of the University of California*

Questions 492–494

Match the following situations with the appropriate legal claim.

(A) Abandonment
(B) Assault
(C) Battery
(D) False imprisonment
(E) Misdiagnosis

492. Informed consent is not obtained for a surgical procedure

493. A physician does not follow up after the acute stage of an illness

494. Restraints are used on a competent, nonviolent patient

Questions 495–497

Match the following actions to the underlying ethical principle.

(A) Autonomy
(B) Beneficence
(C) Euthanasia
(D) Supererogation
(E) Utilitarianism

495. A state legislature decides to allocate funds to prenatal care instead of intensive care nurseries

496. A person with AIDS refuses intubation for *Pneumocystis carinii* pneumonia and dies

497. A 27-year-old woman donates a kidney to her 17-year-old brother who has end-stage renal disease

DIRECTIONS: The group of questions below consists of four lettered headings followed by a set of numbered items. For each numbered item select

A	if the item is associated with	(A) **only**
B	if the item is associated with	(B) **only**
C	if the item is associated with	**both** (A) and (B)
D	if the item is associated with	**neither** (A) nor (B)

Each lettered heading may be used **once, more than once, or not at all.**

Questions 498–500

(A) Claims-made professional liability insurance policy

(B) Occurrence professional liability insurance policy

(C) Both

(D) Neither

498. Events that occurred prior to institution of the policy are covered

499. Amount payable is limited

500. Notification of occurrence and claim is required

Legal and Ethical Issues

Answers

471. The answer is D. *(Rudolph, ed 18. pp 760-764.)* Multiple, 1-cm circular scars may be the result of cigarette burns, an all too common form of child abuse. Retinal hemorrhages can occur from head trauma and also from vigorous shaking back and forth (the "shaken baby syndrome"). Any fracture in a child not yet walking is suspicious for abuse (with the exception of clavicular fractures in neonates and pathologic fractures due to bone disease). Bruises over the shins occur commonly from running and falling and should not in themselves raise suspicions of abuse. Health care personnel are under legal requirements in most states to report suspected child abuse.

472. The answer is D. *(Last, ed 12. pp 1412-1418.)* In three surveys, the frequency of spouse abuse was 3.8 percent (in a national study), 8.5 percent (in Texas), and 10 percent (a Harris poll in Kentucky). Spouse abuse most often occurs in an ongoing pattern. Although patients may present with specific injuries, often complaints are related to injuries incurred in the past and are not recognized by medical personnel as related to spouse abuse. Although alcohol abuse is associated with domestic violence, it seems to be more often the excuse than the cause.

473. The answer is E. *(Centers for Disease Control, State Immunization Requirements for School Children* [*1983*].) All 50 states require proof of immunization against measles, rubella, poliomyelitis, and diphtheria in order for children to attend school, although 6 apply the rule only to new entrants. Immunization against mumps is required in 30 states, against pertussis in 40, and against tetanus in 47 in order to enter school.

474. The answer is B. *(National Center for Health Statistics, pub no 78-1108. pp 3, 48-60, 65.)* The 1978 revision of the U.S. Standard Report of Fetal Death is recommended for state-wide adoption by the National Center for Health Statistics and is designed to collect information that includes the cause of fetal death, demographic data, complications and duration of pregnancy, the weight of the fetus, the characteristics of prenatal care, and labor complications. Some states, because of differing definitions of fetal death, require a fetal death certificate only in cases where gestation has reached the twentieth week; other states require a certificate for all products of conception. While a physician is required to indicate whether an autopsy was performed and, if so, whether the results were used to determine the cause of death, the actual results of an autopsy are not required. In fact, usually a death certificate must be completed by a physician long before autopsy results are available. The weight of the fetus is considered by the Public Health Service to be the primary parameter to allow evaluation of fetal viability.

475. The answer is E. *(Hoekelman, pp 35–38.)* To make an informed decision regarding treatment, patients need to be informed not only of the risks of the treatment, but also of its expected efficacy, and the expected efficacy and risks of alternative treatments. Consent should be obtained before sedation, not only because the discussion should take place while the patient is lucid, but also because sedation itself may be associated with risks. Consent may be obtained verbally. As a general rule, the need to inform patients of adverse effects of treatment is more dependent on the severity of the adverse effect than on its frequency.

476. The answer is A. *(Benenson, ed 15. pp xxiv–xxv.)* The selection of infectious diseases to be reported is usually a matter of local discretion. The reporting of cholera, plague, smallpox, yellow fever, paralytic poliomyelitis, and malaria (as well as viral influenza, louse-borne typhus fever, and louse-borne relapsing fever) is universally required in all countries subject to the 1969 International Health Regulations or agreements at the 22nd World Health Assembly. Because of their potential for causing epidemics, cases of these diseases should be immediately reported to local health authorities.

477. The answer is D. *(Pozgar, ed 4. p 16.)* Legally, negligence is defined in terms of the expected behavior of a "reasonably prudent person" in a certain situation. Criminal negligence is the reckless disregard for the well-being of another and would usually constitute gross negligence as opposed to ordinary negligence. Malpractice is the negligence of a professional person such as a physician, nurse, or lawyer. Malfeasance is the performance of an unlawful act. Misfeasance is the improper performance of a lawful act that results in injury to another.

478. The answer is D. *(Pozgar, ed 4. pp 17–23.)* Duty to use due care is the legal obligation of one party to protect another party by conforming to a specific standard of care. This duty arises from the doctor-patient, nurse-patient or hospital-patient relationship and can be created by a telephone call or by displaying an emergency room sign. A physician passing an accident victim on the highway has a moral obligation to stop and render assistance, but there is no legal obligation because the doctor-patient relationship is not established.

Breach of duty is the failure to fulfill this duty according to the prevailing standard of care. Standard of care is based on the behavior of a hypothetical "reasonably prudent person" with similar training and knowledge. This standard may be a national or an "industry" standard as opposed to a community standard. Expert witness testimony is often used in attempts to define this standard.

Unless injuries actually occur, damages cannot be awarded. Malpractice may have been committed, but if there were no untoward results, damages due to negligence cannot be recovered. The legal term *injuries* includes mental anguish and violation of rights and privileges in addition to physical harm.

Finally, causation must be established. This must be a reasonable and close relationship, but it need not be direct. For example, an accident victim who has never encountered the physician may receive damages for physician negligence when injured by a patient who is driving under the influence of a drug prescribed by the physician if the patient received no warnings concerning the drug's intoxicating nature.

Nonfeasance is a negligent act of omission, failing to perform an act that a reasonably prudent person would be expected to perform under the same circumstances. This would satisfy the criteria for breach of duty, but in itself is not necessary for the awarding of damages.

479.   The answer is C. *(Pozgar, ed 4. pp 261–262.)* Good Samaritan laws free health professionals from ordinary negligence in emergency situations where no preexisting duty to use due care exists. They do not apply to acute situations in the emergency room, but rather are designed to encourage health professionals to volunteer their assistance in emergency situations by eliminating liability concerns. No expectation of financial compensation can exist, for this implies a professional/ contractual relationship. Good Samaritan laws have been enacted by almost all states, but statutes vary; they may apply to laypersons as well. While the laws free providers from liability for ordinary negligence, they do not free persons from liability for gross or criminal negligence or for "willful or wanton" misconduct.

480.   The answer is D. *(Jonsen, ed 2. pp 4–8, 92–94.)* The overriding consideration in questions of clinical ethics is the patient's preference, which reflects the principle of autonomy. In most cases physicians are morally obligated to respect the patient's wishes, and strong efforts to identify the patient's preferences need to be made. Another important general category for consideration is the indication for medical intervention. Physicians need to make objective, educated judgments about the risks and benefits of diagnostic and therapeutic efforts. Measures that clearly are not medically indicated need not be pursued, even in the face of a patient's preference. Examples here include "Do Not Resuscitate" (DNR) orders and termination of ineffective therapy in terminally ill patients. Considerations of quality of life include elements of the patient's preference, disease progression, and efficacy of treatment. If the patient's preferences are known, they are overriding. More often, considerations of quality of life become important in situations where the patient is incompetent to make decisions and no preference has been voiced previously. Economic considerations are becoming more and more important as health care resources become more scarce and decisions are made about the rationing and allocation of health care dollars. These considerations are very important in

expensive, high-technology measures such as organ transplant and intensive care.
The physician's preferences are relatively unimportant in ethical decisions. Objective medical judgment is a critical input as described above, but subjective preference of the physician yields consistently to the patient's preference. However, physicians need not be compelled to act in ways contrary to their own ethical beliefs. For example, an obstetrician cannot be forced to perform abortions or an oncologist forced to provide ongoing chemotherapy for a patient with a terminal, end-stage illness. The physician does, however, have an obligation to assist a patient in finding a new provider who is able to work with the patient.

481.   The answer is E. *(Pozgar, ed 4. pp 165–167.)* The Uniform Anatomical Gift Act permits persons 18 years of age or older to donate their body or parts of their body to medical education, science, or transplantation. The person must be of sound mind and the donation should be made by will or other written instrument. However, if the deceased has made no statements objecting to donation, a donation may still be made if relatives or guardians consent. This consent should be recorded. A donation may be revoked by written or oral means, with specific criteria for witnesses. Persons acting in good faith are not liable for criminal or civil negligence when participating in organ donation unless there has been notice of revocation of donation. This is designed to remove obstacles for participation in organ transplantation procedures and is similar to Good Samaritan laws. To eliminate conflict of interest and the overzealous harvesting of organs, time of death of the donor cannot be certified by any physician involved in the transplant procedure.

482.   The answer is E. *(Jonsen, ed 2. pp 72–79.)* Requirements for competency to refuse or consent to medical treatment include attainment of legal age, the ability to comprehend and communicate information, and the ability to reason and deliberate about one's choices. The legal pronouncement may well require a judicial hearing, which may not be available in clinical emergencies. All the patients portrayed are presumed competent given the available information. Adherence to religious or unusual beliefs does not make one incompetent. Thus, the wishes of the Jehovah's Witness not to be transfused must be respected since they were expressed at a time when she was competent. Change in medical condition does not alter the power of the original statement. Similarly, affective states such as anxiety or (nonpathologic) depression do not make a patient incompetent when he or she refuses recommended medical treatment. One is ethically obligated to work with the patient in this situation and to try to explain options in a comforting manner, but patient autonomy still prevails. The elderly diabetic with a foot ulcer and the executive with chest pain are also competent to refuse medical treatment, for each is capable of understanding information and making a deliberate decision.

483.   The answer is B. *(Rudolph, ed 18. pp 9–10.)* The so-called Baby Doe regulations address the rights of disabled infants. They were developed in the early

182   Preventive Medicine and Public Health

1980s following an instance in which surgical repair of a tracheoesophageal fistula in a newborn infant with Down's syndrome was withheld according to parental wishes. The regulations state that medically indicated treatment will not be withheld from disabled infants with life-threatening conditions except in cases of irreversible coma, in cases in which the treatment only prolongs survival and does not correct the underlying condition, or if treatment is futile and by its nature inhumane. Disabilities that do not preclude an "acceptable" quality of life (for example, Down's syndrome or moderate birth asphyxia) are not in and of themselves sufficient conditions for withholding medical treatment. In contrast, it would be appropriate to withhold treatment for infants with anencephaly, even if the parents desired treatment, since treatment is futile.

484. The answer is E. *(Pozgar, ed 4. pp 28–29, 139–143.)* Physician-patient communication is considered confidential, but is not privileged to the extent of the attorney-client relationship. Violation of this confidentiality is termed *invasion of privacy* and can be cause for damages. However, physicians have specific legally defined reporting obligations which include suspected child abuse, diseases in newborns, certain communicable diseases, births and deaths, suspicious deaths, and gunshot wounds (including those claimed to be accidental). When reporting these conditions in good faith, one is not liable for damages. Substance abuse, to the extent that it does not harm another person, is a confidential communication; such information should not be released without the patient's consent.

485. The answer is E. *(Dorland's Illustrated Medical Dictionary, ed 27. pp 767–768.)* Hippocrates (a late fifth century B.C. Greek) is often regarded as the "Father of Medicine." His oath emphasizes respect for teachers and the obligation to pass knowledge on to the next generation. It is the basis of the pledge to do only good and to do no harm. It specifically forbids active euthanasia, abortion, and the seduction of women or men "be they free or slaves." Substance abuse is not directly mentioned, although he swears "to preserve the purity of my life" and to "prescribe regimen for the good of my patient." Other medical oaths that contribute to the heritage of the physician's ethics include the Daily Prayer of Maimonides (a twelfth century Jewish physician and philosopher) and the Oath of Lasagna (a contemporary American physician).

486. The answer is C. *(Hulley, p 152.)* The DHHS does not require that subjects be compensated for their time or pain. However, some compensation may be helpful in recruiting adequate numbers of subjects for a study. Most importantly, the subjects must understand and must have given informed consent for any risk, inconvenience, or discomfort they will experience as a result of the study. Additional safeguards are required for vulnerable patients, such as prisoners, patients who are mentally incompetent, and children.

487.   The answer is C. *(Kircher, N Engl J Med 313:1263-1269, 1985.)* Because the information recorded on the death certificate is used in determining mortality from various diseases, it is essential that physicians understand how to fill one out. The immediate cause of death (in this case, pulmonary embolism) was not considered to be the condition that was responsible for the death by the attending physician, who determined that the patient died as a result of pancreatic cancer (which caused Trousseau's syndrome, which caused deep venous thrombosis, which resulted in a fatal pulmonary embolism). The last diagnosis listed is recorded in vital statistics; it should be the one that was responsible for setting in motion the chain of events that were eventually fatal.

488.   The answer is D. *(Kircher, N Engl J Med 313:1163-1169, 1985.)* The death certificate has several purposes. It verifies that the patient died and gives the time and place of death and certain demographic information about the deceased. It also indicates the underlying disease that was responsible for the patient's death, so that accurate statistics on disease patterns can be kept. If there are reasons to be concerned about suspicious causes of death (such as poisoning), the physician should contact the coroner. In those cases, the coroner can perform an autopsy at his judgment, even if the family refuses. In this case, as the patient's physician, you attended the death and have no reason to suspect foul play. Breast cancer was the disease that was responsible for her death and *must* be mentioned on the death certificate. Inclusion of the final conditions (cardiac tamponade, pericarditis) is optional. While there may be medical reasons to want an autopsy, it is inappropriate to refuse to sign a death certificate simply to force the family to acquiesce.

489-491.   The answers are: 489-D, 490-E, 491-B. *(Pozgar, ed 4. pp 38-39, 44, 81-82, 189-193.)* Darling v. Charleston Community Memorial Hospital (1965) established hospital liability for the actions of its employees. An 18-year-old football player fractured a leg, was treated in his local hospital over a 2-week period by a general practitioner without specialist consultation, subsequently developed complications, was transferred, and ultimately had a below-the-knee amputation. The physician settled out of court, but the case against the hospital continued charging negligence on a number of grounds, including failure to provide a sufficient number of trained nurses and failure of the nurses to bring the patient's condition to the attention of hospital officials so adequate consultation could be obtained. The hospital was found negligent and liable, thereby establishing the hospital's responsibility for the quality of the patient care administered in the institution. This also established the hospital's responsibility to monitor the credentials and competency of physicians.

The Quinlan case (1976) established that a patient's right to self-determination—and thus to decline medical treatment under certain situations—is protected by the right to privacy. The case involved a 21-year-old woman in a comatose vegetative state whose parents petitioned for the right to refuse treatment and turn off a respirator. The court reached its decision by balancing the state's interest in promoting the sanctity of life against the patient's privacy interest. The father was appointed legal guardian and in accordance with the findings of the hospital ethics committee, the respirator was turned off. Decisions regarding the withdrawal of life support remain very charged and controversial. Clear legal guidelines are still lacking for these decisions and individual decisions need to be made in each case with input from clinicians, ethicists, and often the courts.

Tarasoff v. Regents of the University of California (1976) confirmed the duty to warn. In the course of a psychotherapy session, a therapist was informed of a patient's intention to kill another person. The therapist failed to inform the victim of the patient's intentions, and the victim was subsequently murdered. The court held that the patient's right to privacy did not obviate the therapist's duty to warn possible victims in cases in which a therapist can *reasonably* determine that another person is at *foreseeable* risk. Performance of this duty may include notification of the police.

492–494.   The answers are: 492-C, 493-A, 494-D. *(Pozgar, ed 4. pp 23–25, 59–60.)* Abandonment is the unilateral termination of a doctor-patient relationship by the physician. Abandonment occurs when a physician terminates medical care prematurely (such as failing to follow up after an acute illness), fails to provide adequate cross-coverage, or refuses to see an established patient without notifying the patient and making arrangements to transfer care. The doctor-patient relationship may be ended by mutual consent of both parties, dismissal of the physician by the patient, absence of a requirement for continued medical care, or withdrawal of the physician with notification of the patient. This notification should be written and provide a reasonable transition period.

An assault is a threat to do harm. Battery involves touching another person in a socially unacceptable way without the person's consent. Battery is committed when informed consent is not obtained for medical procedures—diagnostic or therapeutic. The fact that the act may have improved the patient's health is legally irrelevant.

False imprisonment is the illegal confinement or restraint of a person or the illegal restraint of a person's liberty. A competent person who is not allowed to sign out against medical advice or who endures excessive use of physical restraints could sue for false imprisonment. Separate laws govern the involuntary hospitalization of the mentally ill.

495–497.   The answers are: 495-E, 496-A, 497-D. *(Jonsen, ed 2. pp 11–12, 47–51, 129–130, 141–142.)* Utilitarianism is the principle of doing the most good for the most people. It is useful in considering larger policy issues such as allocation of resources, but also applies to individual clinical decisions because in situations where resources are limited, providing care for one person may well mean denying care for another. As a general rule, preventive care will produce greater utility per unit of medical care than will intensive care.

Autonomy is the competent person's moral right to select his or her own course of acton; it is a caveat of medical ethics. The corresponding legal principle is self-determination. A competent person may refuse life-sustaining care and those wishes must be respected. Paternalistic behavior—that is, performing actions in a person's best interests against his or her wishes—is ethically and legally permissible only in very limited situations. The case of the AIDS patient's refusal of intubation illustrates a decision not to progress to further intervention in a fatal disease. It is not an example of "passive" euthanasia, the withdrawal of life-sustaining therapy; nor is it an example of "active" euthanasia, the administration of a lethal agent to end suffering.

A supererogatory act is one beyond the call of duty—one that is morally praiseworthy but cannot be required of a person. No one can claim a corresponding right to the performance of this act. Organ donation, stopping at roadside emergencies, or providing patients with a home phone number could all be acts of supererogation, albeit in decreasing order of importance.

Beneficence is the principle "to do good." Along with nonmalevolence, "to do no harm," it is one of the cornerstones of medical ethics.

498–500.   The answers are: 498-A, 499-C, 500-C. *(Pozgar, ed 4. pp 203–213.)* Professional liability insurance policies (malpractice coverage) include provisions for an insurance agreement, defense and settlement, the policy period, the amount payable, and the conditions of the policy. The policy period varies according to the type of insurance policy. An *occurrence* policy covers all incidents that take place during the year the policy is in effect, regardless of when they are reported or when legal action is initiated (given that the statute of limitations has not expired). Advantages of this form of insurance include continued coverage beyond the time period during which premiums are paid. For example, under this type of policy a retired physician would still be covered for events that occurred during active practice. In contrast, the *claims-made* policy covers only those claims made or reported during the policy year. Insurance companies worry about assuming liability for events that occurred prior to the initiation of the policy, and physicians must worry about ongoing coverage after the policy expires.

Malpractice policies cover professional liability only and contain limitations on the amount of damages covered. Policies usually contain a maximum for any individual claim as well as a limit to aggregate claims. Amounts awarded in excess of the insurance limit must be provided for by the individual professional. The insurance company agrees to provide a defense for the insured against lawsuits in which the attorney's obligations are to the insured professional directly, not to the insurance company. However, insurance companies often retain the power to effect a settlement, in which case the attorney has responsibilities to the insurance company as well.

All insurance policies contain important provisions with which the physician must comply to keep the policy in effect, regardless of the policy period. These include requirements for prompt notification of occurrence and claim and a duty to assist the insurance company to reach a settlement. Other provisions govern relationships with other insurance companies, shared liability, and the terms of change or cancellation of the policy.

Bibliography

Abrams HL, Van Kaenel WE: Medical problems of survivors of nuclear war. *N Engl J Med* 305:1226-1232, 1981.

American Academy of Pediatrics: *Report of the Committee on Infectious Disease*. American Academy of Pediatrics, Evanston, IL, 1988.

Benenson AS (ed): *Control of Communicable Disease in Man*, 15th ed. Washington, DC, American Public Health Association Publications, 1990.

Browner WS, Newman TB: Are all significant p values created equal? The analogy between diagnostic tests and clinical research. *JAMA* 257:2459-2463, 1987.

California Department of Health Services, Infectious Disease Branch: The significance and accuracy of ELISA tests for HIV antibodies. *California Morbidity*, no 44, 1986.

Centers for Disease Control: *Immunization against Disease*. Atlanta, U.S. Department of Health and Human Services, 1983.

Centers for Disease Control: *State Immunization Requirements for School Children*. Atlanta, U.S. Department of Health and Human Services, 1983.

Cherry JD, Brunell PA, Golden GS, Karzon DT: Report of the task force on pertussis and pertussis immunization—1988. *Pediatrics* 81:939-984, 1988.

Colton T: *Statistics in Medicine*. Boston, Little, Brown, 1975.

Croog S, Levine S, Testa M, et al: The effects of antihypertensive therapy on the quality of life. *N Engl J Med* 314:1657-1664, 1986.

Daugherty W, Levi B, Von Hippel F: Casualties due to the blast, heat, and radioactive fallout from various hypothetical nuclear attacks on the United States. In *The Medical Implications of Nuclear War*, Solomon F and Marston RQ, eds. Washington, DC, National Academy Press, 1986, pp 207-232.

Dorland's Illustrated Medical Dictionary, 27th ed. Philadelphia, WB Saunders, 1988.

Ehrlich O, Brem AS: A prospective comparison of urinary tract infections in patients treated with either clean intermittent catheterization or urinary diversion. *Pediatrics* 70:665, 1982.

Expert Panel: Report of the National Cholesterol Education Program Expert Panel on the detection, evaluation and treatment of high blood cholesterol in adults. *Arch Intern Med* 148:37-69, 1988.

Feigin RD, Cherry JD: *Textbook of Pediatric Infectious Disease*, 2d ed. Philadelphia, WB Saunders, 1987.

Freeman HE, Aiken LH, Blendon RJ: Uninsured working-age adults: Characteristics and consequences. *Health Serv Rev* 24:811-823, 1990.

Friedland GH, Klein RS: Transmission of the human immunodeficiency virus. *N Engl J Med* 317:1125–1135, 1987.

Fuchs VR, Hahn JS: How does Canada do it? A comparison of expenditures for physicians' services in the United States and Canada. *N Engl J Med* 323:884–890, 1990.

Gray BH, McNerney MHA: For-profit enterprise in health care: The Institute of Medicine study. *N Engl J Med* 314:1523–1528, 1986.

Greaves WL, Orenstein WA, Hinman AR, et al: Clinical efficacy of rubella vaccine. *Pediatr Infect Dis* 2:284–286, 1983.

Green LW, Anderson CL: *Community Health*, 6th ed. St. Louis, CV Mosby, 1990.

Hearst N, Hulley SB: Preventing the heterosexual spread of AIDS: Are we giving our patients the best advice? *JAMA* 259:2428–2432, 1988.

Hoekelman RA, Blatman S, Friedman SB, et al: *Primary Pediatric Care*. St. Louis, CV Mosby, 1987.

Hulley SB, Cummings S (eds): *Designing Clinical Research: An Epidemiologic Approach*. Baltimore, Williams & Wilkins, 1988.

Igelhart JK: Reducing residency opportunities for graduates of foreign medical schools. *N Engl J Med* 313:831–836, 1985.

Igelhart JK: Early experience with prospective payment of hospitals. *N Engl J Med* 314:1460–1464, 1986.

Ingelfinger JA, Mosteller F, Thibodeau LA, Ware JH: *Biostatistics in Clinical Medicine*, 2d ed. New York, Macmillan, 1987.

Jonsen AR, Siegler M, Winslade WJ: *Clinical Ethics*, 2d ed. New York, Macmillan, 1982.

Kircher T, Nelson J, Burdo H: The autopsy as a measure of accuracy of the death certificate. *N Engl J Med* 313:1263–1269, 1985.

Koonin LM, Atrash HK, Smith HC: Abortion surveillance, 1986–87. *MMWR CDC Surveill Summ* 39:23–56, 1990.

Last JM (ed): *A Dictionary of Epidemiology*, 2d ed. New York, Oxford University Press, 1988.

Last JM: *Maxcy-Rosenau Preventive Medicine and Public Health*, 12th ed. Norwalk, CT, Appleton & Lange, 1986.

LeMasurier J: Physician medical malpractice. *Health Care Financing Review* 7:111–116, 1985.

Lilienfeld AM, Lilienfeld DE: *Foundations of Epidemiology*, 2d ed. New York, Oxford University Press, 1980.

Mandell LA, Ralph ED: *Essentials of Infectious Diseases*. Boston, Blackwell Scientific Publications, 1985.

Mausner JS, Kramer S: *Mausner and Bahn Epidemiology: An Introductory Text*, 2d ed. Philadelphia, WB Saunders, 1985.

Mayer TR, Mayer GG: HMOs: Origins and development. *N Engl J Med* 312:590–594, 1985.

Michael M, Boyce WT, Wilcox AJ: *Biomedical Bestiary: An Epidemiologic Guide to Flaws and Fallacies in the Medical Literature*. Boston, Little, Brown, 1985.

National Center for Health Statistics: *Physicians' Handbook on Medical Certification: Death, Birth, Fetal Death*. Publication No. (PHS) 78-1108. Hyattsville, MD United States Department of Health, Education and Welfare, 1978.

Office of National Cost Estimates: National health expenditures, 1988. *Health Care Financing Review* 11:1-41, 1990.

Pozgar GD: *Legal Aspects of Health Care Administration*, 4th ed. Rockville, MD, Aspen, 1990.

Raffle PAB, Lee WR, McCallum RI, Murray R (eds): *Hunter's Diseases of Occupations*. Boston, Little, Brown, 1987.

Relman AS: The new medical-industrial complex. *N Engl J Med* 303:963-970, 1980.

Rockefeller JD: The Pepper Commission report on comprehensive health care. *N Engl J Med* 323:1004-1007, 1990.

Rosenstock L, Cullen MR: *Clinical Occupational Medicine*. Philadelphia, WB Saunders, 1986.

Rothman KJ: *Modern Epidemiology*. Boston, Little, Brown, 1986.

Rudolph AM, et al (eds): *Pediatrics*, 18th ed. Norwalk, CT, Appleton & Lange, 1987.

Sackett DL, Haynes RB, Tugwell P: *Clinical Epidemiology: A Basic Science for Clinical Medicine*. Boston, Little, Brown, 1985.

Schlesselman JJ, Stolley PD: *Case Control Studies: Design, Conduct, Analysis*. New York, Oxford University Press, 1982.

Siegel AF: *Statistics and Data Analysis: An Introduction*. New York, John Wiley & Sons, 1988.

Stern RS, Epstein AM: Institutional responses to prospective payment based on diagnosis-related groups. Implications for cost, quality, and access. *N Engl J Med* 312:621-627, 1985.

Trunkey DD: Trauma. *Sci Am* 249:28-35, 1983.

United States Preventive Services (USPS) Task Force: *Guide to Clinical Preventive Services: An Assessment of the Effectiveness of 169 Interventions*. Baltimore, Williams & Wilkins, 1989.

Wegman ME: Annual summary of vital statistics—1986. *Pediatrics* 80:817-827, 1987.

Wegman ME: Annual summary of vital statistics—1988. *Pediatrics* 84:943-957, 1989.

Whitney EN, Cataldo CB: *Understanding Normal and Clinical Nutrition*, 2d ed. St. Paul, MN, West Publishing, 1987.

Williams SJ, Torrens PR (eds): *Introduction to Health Services*, 3d ed. New York, John Wiley & Sons, 1988.

Wilson JD, Braunwald E, Isselbacher KJ, et al (eds): *Harrison's Principles of Internal Medicine*, 12th ed. New York, McGraw-Hill, 1991.

Wyngaarden JB, Smith LH Jr: *Cecil Textbook of Medicine*, 18th ed. Philadelphia, WB Saunders, 1988.